Lorraine
on looking great

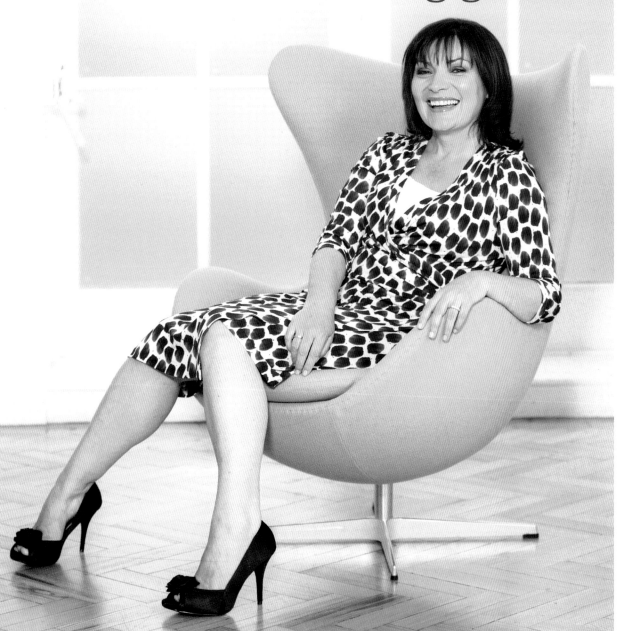

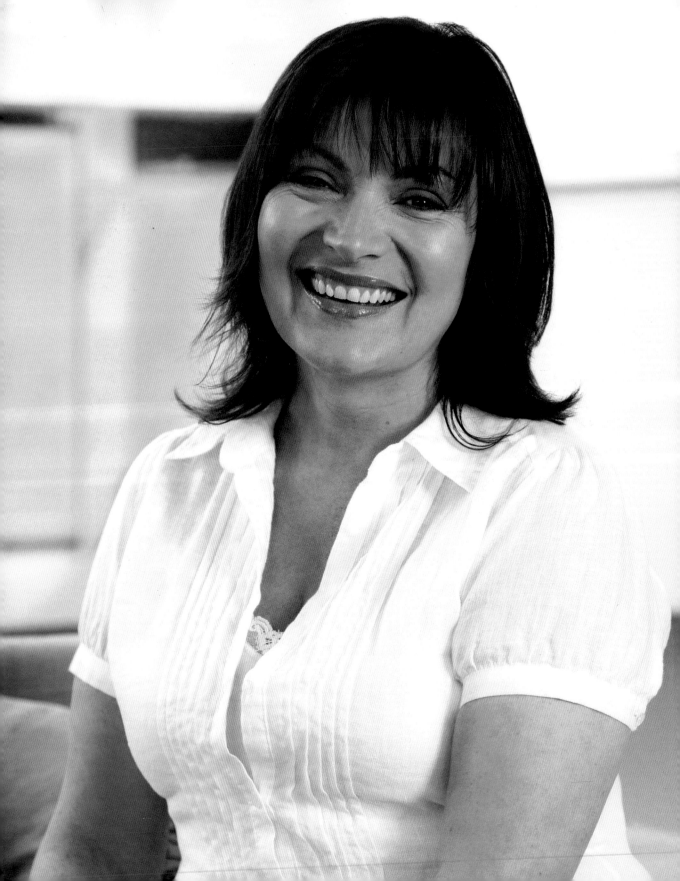

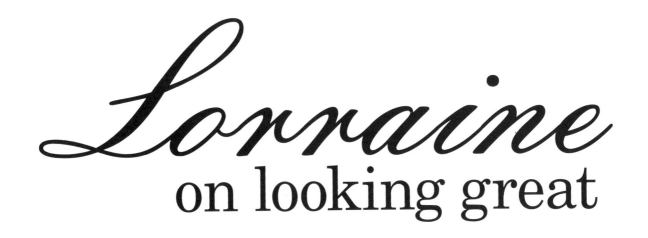

Lorraine
on looking great

my guide for real women

Lorraine Kelly

hamlyn

An Hachette UK Company
www.hachette.co.uk

First published in Great Britain in 2010 by
Hamlyn, a division of Octopus Publishing Group Ltd
Endeavour House
189 Shaftesbury Avenue
London
WC2H 8JG
www.octopusbooks.co.uk

ISBN 978-0-600-61984-0

A CIP catalogue record for this book is available from
the British Library

Printed and bound in China

10 9 8 7 6 5 4 3 2 1

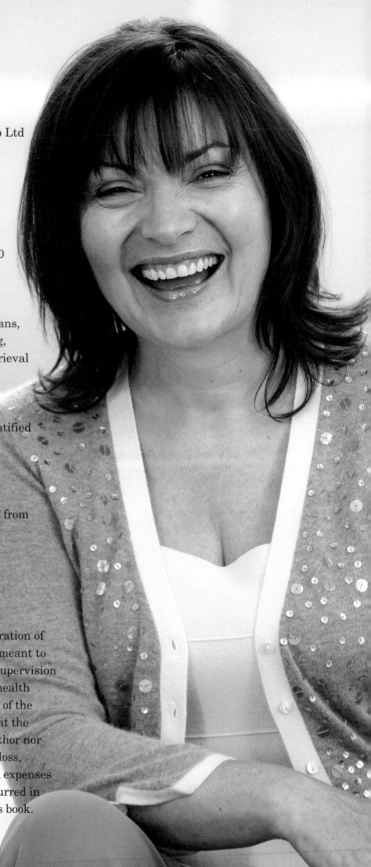

All reasonable care has been taken in the preparation of
this book, but the information it contains is not meant to
take the place of medical care under the direct supervision
of a doctor. Before making any changes in your health
regime, always consult a doctor. Any application of the
ideas and information contained in this book is at the
reader's sole discretion and risk. Neither the author nor
the publisher will be responsible for any injury, loss,
damages, actions, proceedings, claims, demands, expenses
and costs (including legal costs or expenses) incurred in
any way arising out of following exercises in this book.

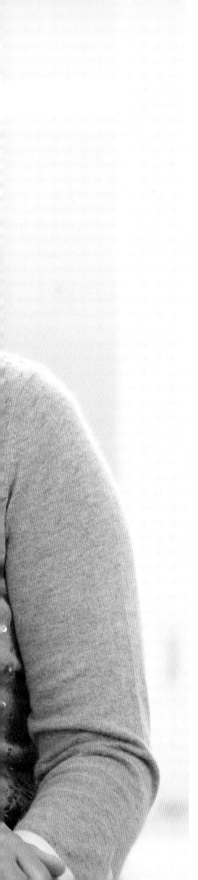

Contents

Introduction

THIS BOOK IS ALL ABOUT LOOKING GOOD AND FEELING GREAT. I WANT TO SHARE WITH YOU THE EXPERT ADVICE AND INFORMATION THAT I HAVE RECEIVED OVER THE YEARS AND USE WHAT I HAVE LEARNED TO HELP YOU FEEL HAPPIER, HEALTHIER AND MORE CONFIDENT.

my weight has gone up and down over the years, like most women, but I have finally realized that yo-yo dieting is not the answer. Instead of yearning for an impossibly slim body, I am now comfortable with the shape and size that I am meant to be. I focus on eating healthily and have turned my back on those faddy diets that only work in the short term and that might even result in my being bigger and more miserable than I was in the first place.

More importantly I have discovered that, in order to get into shape, you really have to combine a healthy eating plan with some exercise. I always used to make the excuse that I didn't have the time to exercise – until my husband pointed out that I managed to find the time to watch my favourite soap four or five times a week. I realized if I could find time to watch television, then surely I could fit in half an hour of exercise almost every day. But this didn't mean hiring a personal trainer, wearing expensive designer sportswear or spending hours in the gym, I simply made sure that I went for a brisk walk with my dog Rocky most days and I joined a Pilates class once a week. I have stuck to these changes and they have made a huge difference to my fitness.

Over the years, as many of you will know, I have committed some truly terrible crimes against fashion and, looking back, some of my hairstyles have been quite hideous. But I have learned from my mistakes, and look better today than I did in the 80s simply by dressing in clothes that suit me, having a great haircut and using make-up to my advantage. You can do this too.

Looking and feeling good is about much more than what's happening on the outside with hairdos, clothes and make-up, however, and that's why I like to stay well informed about health issues such as breast cancer and osteoporosis. This way I can do the right things to protect and take care of myself as I grow older.

The following pages offer a wealth of useful information for getting into shape. You'll find all the facts about eating well, essential health advice and beauty and style tips, plus a safe, but effective, weight-loss plan and an exercise regime to help get you started.

WHATEVER YOUR AGE OR YOUR LIFESTYLE, YOU'LL FIND SOMETHING IN THIS BOOK THAT WILL HELP YOU TO MAKE THE MOST OF YOURSELF.

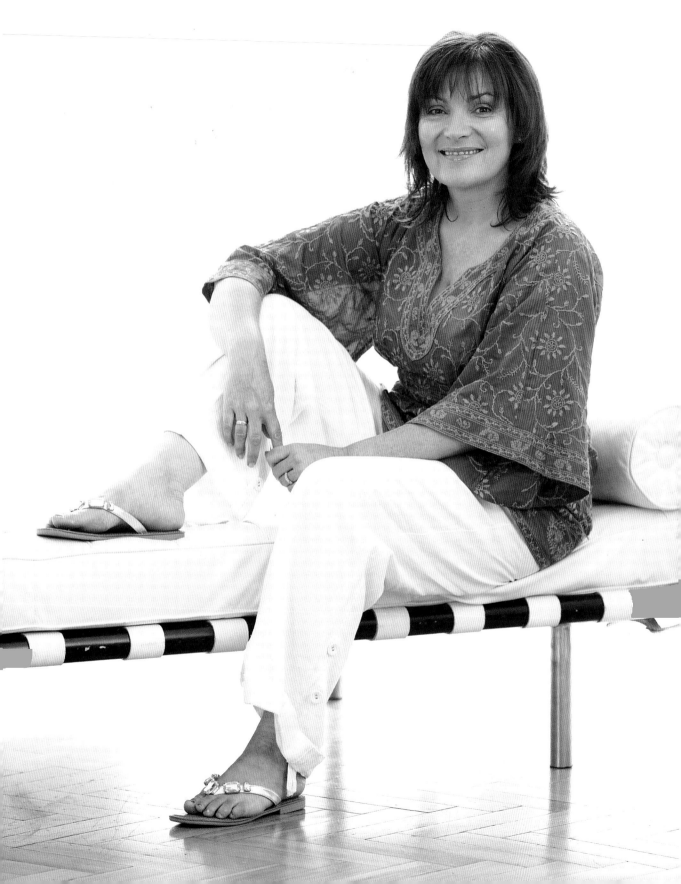

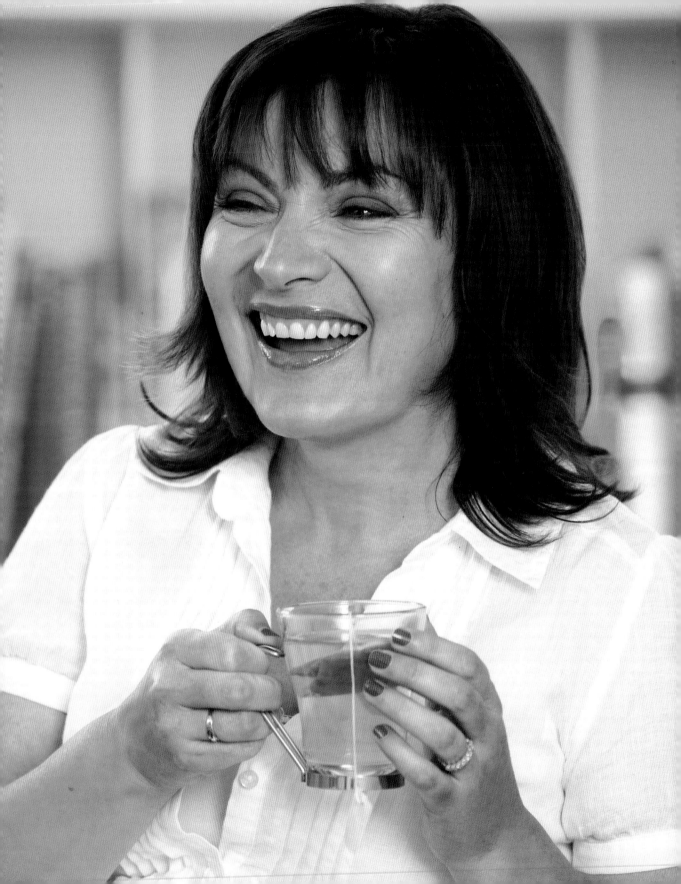

HEALTHY EATING

Food as fuel

AT TIMES, I FIND MYSELF UTTERLY BEMUSED
AS TO WHAT EXACTLY CONSTITUTES A
HEALTHY DIET. ONE WEEK WE ARE WARNED
ABOUT THE DANGER OF DRINKING MORE
THAN A COUPLE OF GLASSES OF WINE AND
THE NEXT WEEK WE ARE TOLD THAT RED
WINE CAN PREVENT HEART DISEASE.

this is confusing and intensely irritating – especially if, like me, you are trying to make sure you and your family are eating well. Take my advice: don't panic and react unquestioningly to every health scare. An occasional bacon sandwich is not going to give you cancer and you are not a bad mother if you have a glass of wine now and again. The key to eating well is to eat a varied diet that focuses on foods that positively fuel your body, while limiting those that lack nutrients or do your body harm.

In order to thrive, your body needs a range of foods that fall into four basic groups. Without some level of each of them in your daily diet you will struggle to reach your optimum health.

CARBOHYDRATES

These are the foods that most easily supply energy to your body. They include bread, rice, pasta and starchy vegetables like potatoes. When you eat a carbohydrate, it is digested by your body and turned into a sugar called glucose, which you use for fuel. However, some carbohydrates – often, refined versions of foods like bread or cereal – are digested quickly by your body, causing a rapid influx of sugar into your system. This triggers your body to release hormones to redress the balance by removing the sugar. The result is an energy crash,

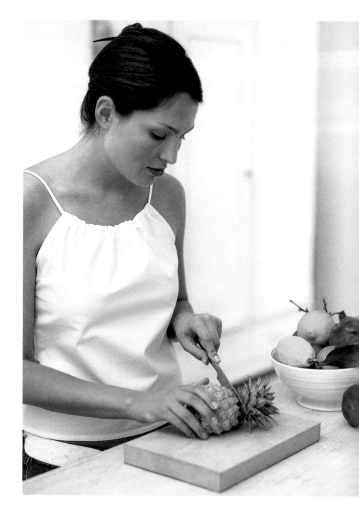

which often sees you craving more sugar for a boost. These foods are known as high glycaemic index (GI) foods and should be eaten sparingly.

Instead, the majority of your carbohydrates should be low GI foods, which are digested slowly and supply a steady flow of energy to fuel you more effectively. These foods are generally unrefined and high in fibre; good examples include granary or rye breads, porridge, oats, all pastas, basmati rice and grains like barley and bulgar wheat. Carbohydrates should make up around 50 per cent of your daily calories.

PROTEIN

This is the nutrient your body uses to fuel its repair and regeneration. If protein levels in your diet are low, this will quickly show in the condition of your hair and nails. Animal products like meat, fish, poultry, dairy and eggs supply the highest levels of protein per gram as well as all eight of the essential amino acids you need to get from your diet each day, but you can also get protein from non-animal sources such as beans, lentils, nuts, soya and Quorn™. In fact, the healthiest way to get your protein is by eating a mixture of meat and non-meat meals each week. Ideally your body needs two small portions of, preferably low-fat, protein a day.

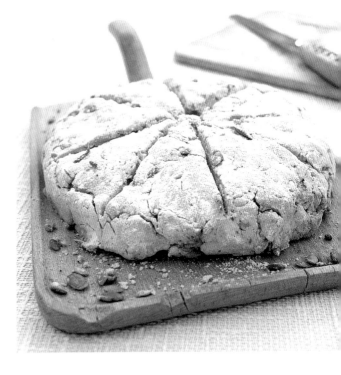

development and function, but also seem to boost mood and heart health. Women of childbearing age should aim for up to two portions of oily fish a week, while women past childbearing age can eat as many as three or four.

HEALTHY FATS

Without a little fat in your diet, you can't absorb fat-soluble vitamins such as A, D and E and your hormone levels can become unbalanced. However you do have to choose the right kinds of fat, known as unsaturated fat. Generally this comes from vegetable sources like nuts, seeds and olives or from oily fish. They are more easily used by your body and supply health-boosting ingredients, such as the omega-3 fats found most readily in oily fish. These are essential for brain

LOAD UP THE CUPBOARD AND FREEZER WITH FRUIT AND VEGETABLES FOR THOSE TIMES THAT YOU CAN'T GET TO THE SUPERMARKET

FRUIT AND VEGETABLES

You need at least five portions of these every day. Not only do fruit and vegetables provide you with vitamins and minerals they also supply compounds called phytochemicals, which appear to have endless disease-fighting and anti-ageing properties. Phytochemicals are found in the pigment that gives the skin and flesh of plants their colour, and you should choose differently coloured fruit and vegetables for the best possible mix. And don't forget: fresh, frozen, dried and canned fruit can all be equally

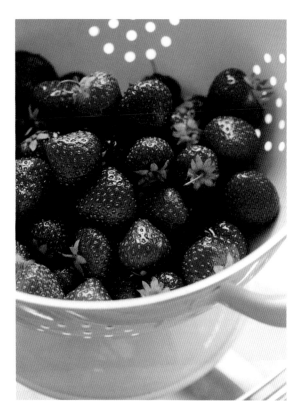

It's generally recommended that you get 24 g of fibre a day. You'll achieve this easily if you eat at least five portions of fruit and vegetables, stick to wholegrain carbohydrates and regularly use beans and pulses in your meals.

VITAMINS AND MINERALS

Your body needs a total of 13 vitamins and 22 minerals each day, all of which help to fuel everything from bone growth to energy levels. Here's a quick guide to the main players:

Vitamin A Found in liver, oily fish and egg yolks, as well as orange, yellow and dark green vegetables, vitamin A is important for growth, good skin and eye health. The recommended intake for women is 600 micrograms (mcg) a day. Vitamin A can be toxic in high doses so don't overload on sources like liver and avoid high-dose vitamin A supplements.

B vitamins The six B vitamins are B1 (thiamin),

good for you – just make sure you avoid versions with added salt or sugar (see 'How to eat five', pages 14–15).

A HIGH-FIBRE DIET

Found in fruit, vegetables, beans, pulses and wholegrain carbohydrates such as bran and oats, fibre is what gives these foods their bulk and texture, and while your body doesn't actually absorb it, fibre provides a myriad of health benefits as it passes through your system. The best-known of these is that of keeping your bowels regular, which in turn helps to reduce problems like bloating, gas and other digestive upsets. Fibre has also been shown to reduce cholesterol and may be linked to a lower risk of some cancers including those of the breast and bowel. Finally, fibre can be linked to weight loss. Not only does a high-fibre diet fill you up more effectively than a low-fibre one, but fibre also blocks the absorption of some of the fat, protein and carbohydrate calories you eat.

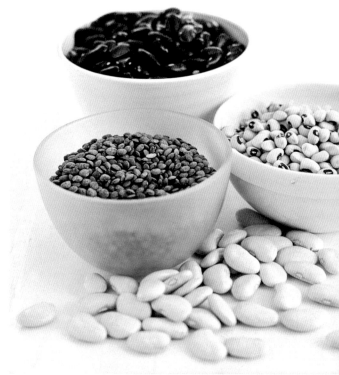

B2 (riboflavin), B3 (nicotinic acid), B6 (pyridoxine), B12 (cobalamin) and folate (folic acid). Their primary jobs are to convert food into energy, to increase immunity and to maintain a healthy nervous system. Because all the B vitamins work together, it's best to focus on thinking of them as a whole group rather than in individual doses. Eating plenty of whole grains, lean meats, dairy produce, green vegetables and dried fruit will ensure a healthy intake. Recommended intake of B vitamins for women is as follows: B1: 0.8 mg; B2: 1.1 mg; B3: 13 mg; B6: 1.2 mcg; B12: 1.5 mcg; folate 200 mcg.

Vitamin C Very important in aiding immune function and wound healing, vitamin C is found in high doses in citrus fruit, blueberries, red peppers and potatoes. The minimum amount you need each day is 40 mg – you can get that in a large orange.

Vitamin D Also known as the sunshine vitamin because the skin makes it when hit by ultraviolet (UV) rays, vitamin D is known to boost immunity and bone health – and is now potentially being linked to cancer prevention. Good food sources include oily fish and dairy products, but most of us get what we need by spending a little time outside in the sun with our hands and face exposed.

Vitamin E Good for the heart, the skin and the brain, vitamin E is found in foods high in healthy fats, such as avocados, nuts and seeds. You'll also find it blackberries, wheat germ and mangoes. A dose of 3–4 mg a day is linked to good heart health.

Calcium Vital for healthy bones and teeth, the best source of calcium is in dairy products, such as milk, yogurt and cheese. You'll also find high levels in foods like tofu, fish with soft bones (canned salmon or sardines) and green leafy vegetables like spinach. You need around 700 mg of calcium a day.

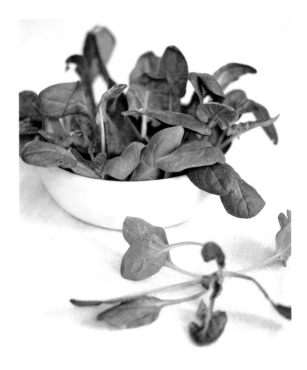

> THE BODY IS LIKE A COMPLICATED MACHINE – IT NEEDS THE RIGHT BALANCE OF CARBOHYDRATES, PROTEIN, FAT, VITAMINS AND MINERALS TO RUN SMOOTHLY AND EFFICIENTLY

Iron Important for healthy blood, good immunity and muscle growth, the best source of iron is red meat because it contains the form we find easiest to absorb. Other sources include dark green vegetables (such as spinach, broccoli and watercress), egg yolks, oily fish and beans – but you have to eat very high doses of these foods to get the recommended 14.8 mg you need each day.

Zinc Another vital immunity-boosting nutrient, zinc is also involved in fertility. It's recommended that you get 15 mg a day, with foods like shellfish, brown rice and nuts/seeds being good sources.

Magnesium Involved in bone health, hormone regulation and potentially good for the heart, magnesium-rich foods include wholegrain cereals, nuts and seeds, yogurt and dried fruit. You need around 270 mg a day.

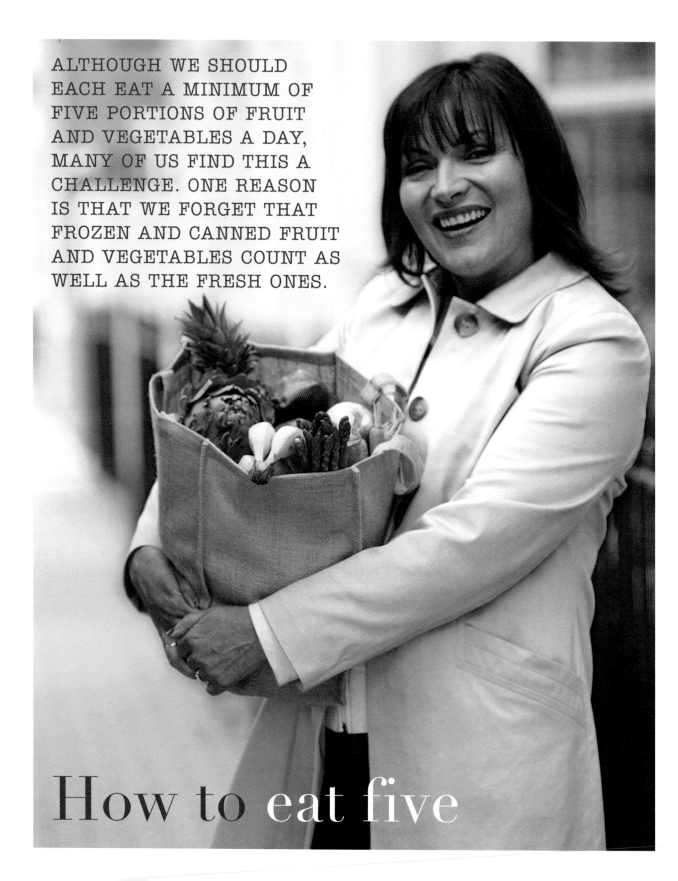

ALTHOUGH WE SHOULD EACH EAT A MINIMUM OF FIVE PORTIONS OF FRUIT AND VEGETABLES A DAY, MANY OF US FIND THIS A CHALLENGE. ONE REASON IS THAT WE FORGET THAT FROZEN AND CANNED FRUIT AND VEGETABLES COUNT AS WELL AS THE FRESH ONES.

How to eat five

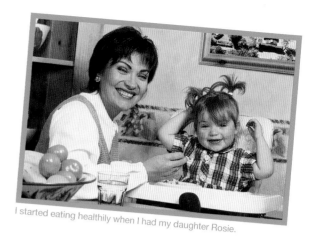

I started eating healthily when I had my daughter Rosie.

actually knowing what makes a 'portion' is vital. This makes it easy to build up your daily intake. The box below shows how much fruit and vegetables you need to make a single portion of your five a day.

BOOST YOUR INTAKE

Now that you know what makes a portion, it should be easy to mix and match juices, smoothies and whole fruits and vegetables to get your five a day. A good tip is to have one portion at breakfast time, two at lunch and two at dinner. If you still think you might struggle, take some tips from me:

Grate, chop, sprinkle Fruit and vegetables can add bulk to soups, stews, sandwiches and more. Sprinkle a chopped apple into your muesli in the morning; add 2 tablespoons of chopped carrots to a prepared soup for lunch; or add 2 tablespoons of Brussels sprouts to your supper-time mashed potato. That's three servings already!

Have a starter or dessert Starting your meal with a small salad adds another portion to your day and may prevent you overeating at your main meal. Or finish with a healthy fruit dessert, such as poached pear, to satisfy sweet cravings.

Get adventurous Citrus fruit can liven up salads. Apples work brilliantly in Asian stir-fries, while avocado or grilled/canned tomatoes on toast work well for breakfast. Try things out.

Think variety Eat lots of different types of food. Instead of a big pile of broccoli, go for a small portion plus a second one of sweetcorn. Not only does this look less daunting, but it offers variety and doubles the phytonutrients you're exposed to.

Keep fruit and vegetables in view You are nearly three times more likely to eat a food if it's on the middle shelf of your refrigerator than anywhere else.

FRUIT

One portion =

1 large slice of a large fruit (melon, pineapple)

1 medium fruit (apple, orange, banana)

2 small fruits (apricot, kiwifruit, tomato)

1 mugful of berries (strawberries, blueberries, cherries)

3 tablespoons of stewed or canned fruit

1 tablespoon of dried fruit

VEGETABLES

One portion =

1 dessert bowlful of light-coloured salad vegetables (cucumber, iceberg lettuce)

2 tablespoons of other vegetables

½ mugful of beans and pulses (only one serving counts towards a day's portions)

½ mugful of vegetable sauces/ dips (fresh tomato pasta sauce or salsa)

Note: potatoes do not count towards your five a day.

JUICES AND SMOOTHIES

One portion =

150 ml (¼ pint) fruit and vegetable juice (only one serving counts towards a day's portions)

Because you use whole fruit in smoothies (and not just their juice), each addition counts as a portion. For example, a smoothie containing a banana, a glass of fruit juice and a mugful of berries will count as three portions in one glass.

Know your enemy

NOW THAT YOU KNOW WHICH FOODS FUEL YOUR BODY, IT'S TIME TO INTRODUCE THE ONES THAT CAN DO POTENTIAL HARM. THESE FOODS SHOULD BE LIMITED IN A HEALTHY DIET.

SATURATED FATS

These fats are linked to raised levels of cholesterol, furring of the arteries and potentially the development of cancer. They are most commonly found in animal products and hard margarines (and items made from them, such as biscuits, cakes and pastry) and you can lower your intake by trimming obvious fat from fresh meat, avoiding processed meats, which often contain high levels, and choosing reduced-fat versions of margarine and dairy goods whenever you can. Ideally you should consume no more than 20 g of saturated fat daily.

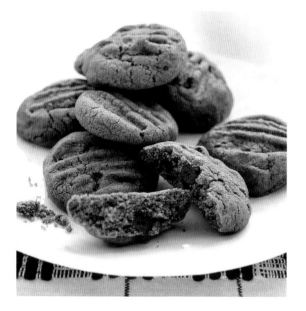

SUGAR

Sugar supplies no healthy nutrients to your body. Instead it produces high levels of ageing free radicals and triggers the production of heart-harming triglycerides in your blood. On top of this, high-sugar diets are linked to obesity, depression, lowered immunity and poor skin. About 40 g of sugar a day is seen as a safe level – that's roughly 10 teaspoons. You might think that this is easy to achieve, but you should be aware that sugar is found in a large number of processed foods. For example, half a can of baked beans can contain 3 teaspoons, and a serving of pasta sauce 2 teaspoons of sugar.

ARTIFICIAL SWEETENERS

While the debate continues as to whether these can be linked to cancer in humans, studies do seem to show that they confuse our bodies when it comes to weight loss. In trials at Tufts University in Boston, Massachusetts, rats given yogurt with sweeteners gained a lower rise in body temperature than those eating yogurt with real sugar, meaning they didn't burn off the kilojoules they'd consumed as quickly.

SALT

Most of us need to reduce our salt consumption by about one-third to in order to reach the government's recommended limit of 6 g a day. Salt is known to raise blood pressure, which increases

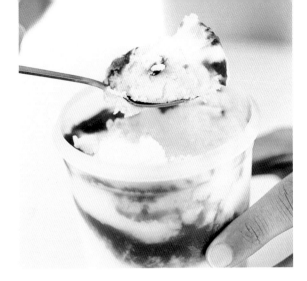

the risk of heart disease and stroke. It has been estimated that, if every single one of us cut our salt intake to that 6 g, some 70,000 strokes and heart attacks would be prevented every year. Stop adding salt to your food at the table or during cooking, and look out for low-salt products when shopping – the majority of our salt intake comes from processed foods like bread, soup, ready meals and even breakfast cereals.

READ YOUR LABELS

Labels tell you all there is to know about what is contained in the food you are buying. The first things to look at are the calories and fat content.

VITAMIN SUPPLEMENTS

Every nutrition guru will tell you that vitamin supplements can't replace fresh food, but that doesn't mean that there aren't some benefits. New research has shown that the parts of cells called telomeres, which determine how fast we age, are healthier in people who take multivitamins. The best advice is to take them if you can afford them, but make sure you use them to boost a healthy diet and not to replace it. If you do take them, be sure to choose reputable supplements that are well constructed with the forms of nutrients your body can best absorb.

Take care, however, as many companies label these per serving – and their servings may differ from yours. Another important factor is the order of the ingredients, which are always listed by weight: the higher up the list an item is, the more there is of it in the product. Finally, there are some things you don't want to see on a label of any food you eat:

Hydrogenated fats Also known as transfats, these are most commonly found in cheap margarines and foods made from them. They've been linked to heart disease and many experts say they're even more dangerous than saturated fats. Most companies are currently phasing them out.

High fructose corn syrup This sweetener sometimes appears under the name glucose-fructose syrup. It has been linked to diabetes and an increased risk of obesity. As well as adding calories to a food, once in your system it may interfere with your appetite, suppressing hormones and encouraging overeating.

E numbers These are added to foods to boost colour, flavour or shelf life. Many of them are harmless, but others have been linked to behaviour issues in children. Check with the UK Food Standards Agency for the main offenders.

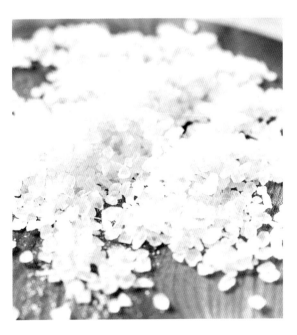

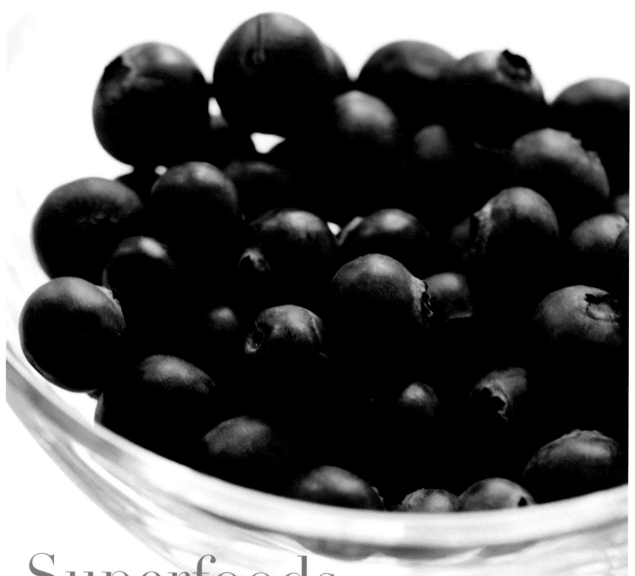

Superfoods

THE MOST IMPORTANT ASPECT OF
HEALTHY EATING IS EATING FOOD THAT
YOU ENJOY. AMONG THOSE FOODS ARE
LIKELY TO BE SOME THAT ARE SHAPING UP
TO HAVE SUCH HIGH LEVELS OF HEALTH-
GIVING PROPERTIES THAT THEY ARE BEING
CALLED 'SUPERFOODS'.

MY FAVOURITE SUPERFOODS

Here's a list of my favourites, along with an idea of what can they do for you:

Apples One of the top superfoods for helping you live longer, apples are a great source of fibre and are packed with antioxidants. Red apples are more potent than green.

Beans A great source of both protein and fibre. Eating beans at least four times a week lowers your risk of heart disease by as much as 22 per cent. They may also lower the risk of colon and breast cancer.

Blueberries Packed with vitamin C, blueberries are among those fruits with the highest levels of antioxidants. They've also been shown to help your brain cells talk to each other.

Broccoli Proven to fight tumour growth and reverse deterioration of your immune system as you age, broccoli also contains vitamin K, which builds bones.

Dark chocolate Another antioxidant, dark chocolate also includes circulation-boosting ingredients. It is high in calories though, so remember that four squares is the ideal health-boosting 'dose'.

Fish The best source of heart- and brain-boosting omega-3 fats, oily fish such as salmon, herring, sardines or trout also contain vitamin D, which is linked to bone health, immunity and lowered risk of cancer.

Mushrooms These contain more antioxidants than green peppers or pumpkins, give you a dose of anti-ageing vitamin D and actively improve the bug-killing power of your immune system.

Nuts Associated with a lower risk of heart disease, lower weight and basically all-round good health, nuts are also a good source of omega-3 fats, vitamin E and minerals like magnesium.

Oats These contain many minerals and vitamin E. Their secret weapon, however, is a fibre called beta glucan, which is shown to lower cholesterol and stimulate the immune system.

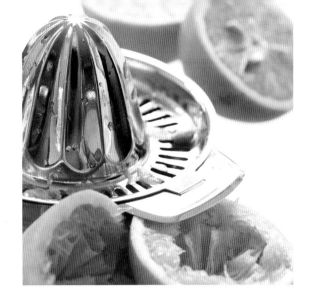

Oranges Not only do oranges contain vitamin C and fibre, but they're one of the few sources of a powerful antioxidant called hesperidin, which may have cancer-fighting potential.

Pomegranate juice This lowers cholesterol, decreases blood pressure and contains more antioxidants than red wine, broccoli or green tea.

Red wine This contains an antioxidant called resveratrol, which is currently linked to a lowered risk of heart disease and some cancers. Remember, however, that no more than 1–2 units of alcohol a day is recommended.

Soya A great protein source, soya contains ingredients called phytoestrogens. These hormone-like substances are linked to better bone health and possibly a lower risk of some cancers.

Tea Among its many health-boosting attributes tea has been shown to reduce stress, fight dental decay and boost immunity.

Tomatoes The best source of the antioxidant, lycopene – linked to a lower risk of cancer and heart disease and eye health – tomatoes are also a good source of potassium.

Yogurt As well as containing protein and calcium, yogurt has healthy bacteria called probiotics. These help your digestive system but are also involved in healthy immunity.

> EAT FOODS THAT YOU ENJOY SO THAT IT BECOMES A HEALTHY HABIT FOR LIFE

Veggies and vegans

WITH ALL THE SCARE STORIES ABOUT CURED
MEAT AND THE TERRIFYING PROSPECT OF THE
HUMAN FORM OF MAD COW DISEASE (BSE)
INFECTING OUR POPULATION, AT ONE POINT IT
DID LOOK LIKELY THAT VEGETARIANISM WAS
THE ONLY WAY FORWARD.

While there have, sadly, been too many victims of Creutzfeldt-Jakob disease (CJD), the projected epidemic has, so far, failed to materialize, but I can understand why, for ethical or health reasons, many people opt for a vegetarian lifestyle. I am concerned, however, that many young girls think that cutting out meat and replacing meals with bowls of cereal will keep them healthy – obviously it won't.

IT IS PERFECTLY POSSIBLE TO EAT NO MEAT, FISH OR DAIRY PRODUCTS AND BE HEALTHY

When you start to cut food groups out of a diet, you increase your chances of developing nutritional deficiencies. The good news is that it is perfectly possibly to eat no meat, fish or dairy products and remain healthy – but only if you take extra care. Here are the most important rules:

Watch your fat levels While a well-constructed vegetarian diet is low in fat, many new vegetarians rely too heavily on cheese and other dairy products. Experiment with low-fat protein sources, such as Quorn™, tofu, tempe (tofu-like cake) and textured vegetable protein (TVP). Seek out vegan cheeses and meat alternatives to add variety.

Use the complete proteins For optimum health, your body needs to get eight essential amino acids from the foods you eat. While animal proteins contain all of these of these, vegetable-based proteins generally don't. The exceptions to this are soya and Quorn™, so eat these regularly. Non-vegans should also include low-fat cheese, milk, yogurt and eggs.

Combine correctly In order to get the eight amino acids from other vegetable foods, you need to combine different types of vegetable protein. For example, eat grains (rice, bread, cereals) together with pulses (lentils, beans); pulses with nuts; or

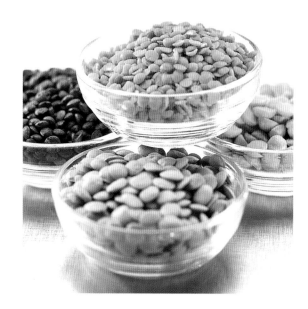

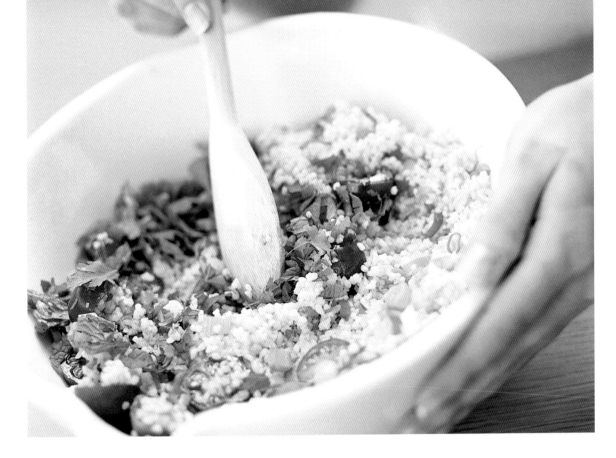

nuts with grains. It used to be thought that you had to do this for every meal, but it's now known that it is sufficient to eat a mix of these foods throughout the day. Easy examples that offer perfect combinations are baked beans on toast, bean chilli with rice or lentil soup.

Watch your iron levels Although dark-green leafy vegetables, egg yolks and wholegrain cereals include iron, your body finds it harder to absorb iron from these foods than from meat. Combine iron-rich foods with a source of vitamin C, which increases iron absorption threefold, or with orange foods, such as carrots or sweet potatoes, which contain betacarotene and double the iron uptake.

Seek out B12 This nutrient is only found in animal products. You don't want much each day, but it is essential, and vegans should take particular care. You need 3 mcg daily, from fortified foods like cereals or soya milk. Alternatively, you can take 10 mcg a day in supplement form.

FOOD ALLERGIES AND INTOLERANCE

Allergies and intolerance are common reasons for people cutting particular foods out of their diet. While 1–2 per cent of the population has an allergy to certain foods (which tend to manifest in rashes, itching or facial swelling) and should always be treated by total exclusion of those foods, some 20 per cent of us could be suffering from food intolerances, which result in symptoms such as bloating, nausea, headaches, diarrhoea, skin irritation or fatigue.

The problem is that many of us diagnose problem foods for ourselves, cutting out things at random. This is a bad idea, as it is all too easy to misdiagnose the problem. For example, you might think that you are intolerant to wheat and cut out all wheat products, when the root of the problem could be a preservative used in the brand of bread you normally buy. Therefore, if you think you have food intolerance, you should see your GP and get a test to confirm it.

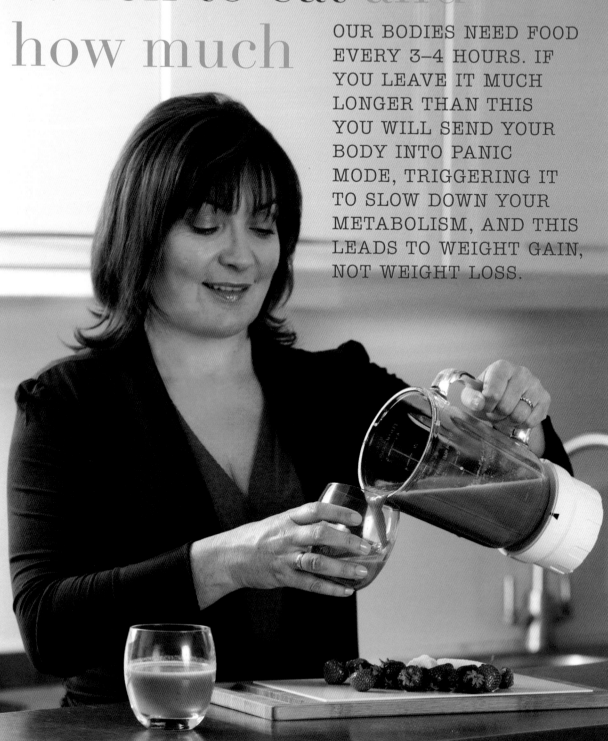

When to eat and how much

OUR BODIES NEED FOOD EVERY 3–4 HOURS. IF YOU LEAVE IT MUCH LONGER THAN THIS YOU WILL SEND YOUR BODY INTO PANIC MODE, TRIGGERING IT TO SLOW DOWN YOUR METABOLISM, AND THIS LEADS TO WEIGHT GAIN, NOT WEIGHT LOSS.

as general rule, most people need to eat three main meals and one or two snacks a day. However, the amount of food you eat at each of these meals is very important. Experts say that one of the main reasons we're getting bigger is not so much *what* we're eating, but *how much* of it we consume. We are living in a supersize society – serving plates have grown one-third bigger over the years. Also, the more we eat out, the more we become used to huge 'value for money' portions, which we then start to serve ourselves when we get home. Controlling portion size can help you rebalance your eating, and there are a couple ways of doing this.

THE SUPER-SPECIFIC APPROACH

Controlling your weight is basically a matter of eating fewer calories than you burn up each day. Therefore the most specific way to calculate how much you can eat each day is to work out how many calories you burn. You can do this by multiplying your weight in pounds by a certain factor depending on how sedentary your lifestyle is (see box). This will give you the daily number of calories that you can consume without putting on weight. By weighing and measuring your portions, you will then be able to tailor-make your own eating plan – keeping a food diary (see page 37) will help here.

THE EYEBALL METHOD

This is the method many nutritionists recommend, as it naturally balances your food intake without becoming obsessive over numbers. The method also pretty much ensures that you'll reach all the healthy nutritional guidelines discussed on pages 10–13. The idea is that, at each meal, you fill half your plate with vegetables or fruit, then add a portion of healthy carbohydrates – roughly the size of your clenched fist – and a portion of protein

about the thickness and diameter of the palm of your hand. An additional serving of healthy fat, about the size of the top joint of your thumb, provides a meal that is perfectly balanced.

SNACK ATTACKS – YES OR NO?

Snacking has a bad reputation but, in fact, in a world in which the gap between lunch and getting home at night could be 7–8 hours, it's vital to keep up your energy and boost your metabolism. Snackers who choose healthy options also increase their intake of nutrients and are more likely to reach their five fruit and vegetables a day (see pages 14–15). The perfect snack is around 100 calories and contains a little protein and some fruit or vegetables (good choices are yogurt and fruit, crudités and hummus.). Having said this, it would be a sad world indeed if you didn't get a treat occasionally, so if the rest of your diet is good, allow yourself to spend your snack on something totally indulgent – a favourite bar of chocolate or a bag of potato crisps – once or twice a week. Remember, there's no such thing as a bad food, only a bad diet.

> THE PERFECT SNACK IS AROUND 100 CALORIES AND CONTAINS A LITTLE BIT OF PROTEIN AND SOME FRUIT OR VEGETABLES

HOW MANY CALORIES DO YOU BURN?

To find out how many calories you burn on a daily basis, calculate your weight in pounds and multiply this by one of the following factors:

- By 12, if you have a sedentary job and do no exercise or only exercise gently.
- By 13, if you have a sedentary job but exercise intensely (more than walking) for at least 30 minutes most days.
- By 15, if you are very active during the day and/or exercise intensely for at least an hour most days.

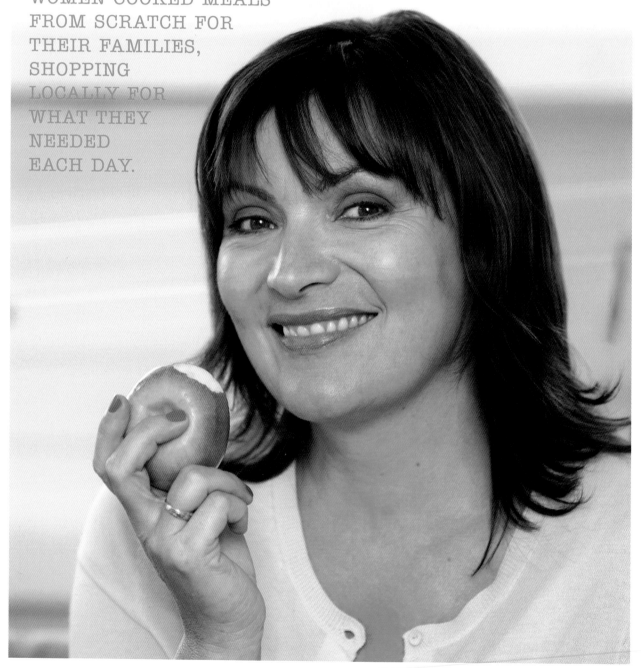

In the kitchen

IN THE OLD DAYS IT WAS EASY, MOST DIETS
DEPENDED ON THE CHANGING SEASONS AND
WOMEN COOKED MEALS
FROM SCRATCH FOR
THEIR FAMILIES,
SHOPPING
LOCALLY FOR
WHAT THEY
NEEDED
EACH DAY.

these days, most families do a massive weekly supermarket shop, stuffing their trolleys with things they don't need and spending a fortune on ready meals and sugary snacks.

As a working mum, I know just how difficult it is to find the time to do a daily shop and make a home-cooked meal – but the benefits are tremendous. Of course, there's no point buying all manner of healthy, nutritious foods, if you then turn them into unhealthy foods by cooking them badly. Here are my tips for healthy cooking:

Keep it crunchy The longer you cook your vegetables the more nutrients they lose. This is particularly the case if you boil them, as the nutrients easily transfer into the cooking water. Ideally, steam, griddle or microwave your vegetables, and eat with a little crunch to them. If you do boil them, use the water as the base for gravy to avoid losing the nutrients altogether.

Don't peel Much of the fibre found in fruit and vegetables is in the skin. Many of the vegetables we traditionally peel (carrots or potatoes) can be eaten with skins on after a good wash.

Grill, poach, steam These methods for cooking meat and fish are preferable to frying or roasting, because they don't require you to add extra fat for cooking.

Fry lightly If you are pan-frying, whenever possible, use an oil spray, ideally of a healthy fat like olive oil – instead of pouring oil into the pan. These give enough oil to stop food sticking to the pan but add only 1–2 calories and virtually no saturated fat. Avoid deep-fat frying altogether.

Mix and match The idea that all vegetables are more nutritious raw is a myth – some actually release higher levels of nutrients if they are cooked – carrots and tomatoes particularly. The healthy approach is to mix cooked and raw vegetables according to taste and season.

Go easy on the barbecue Avoid char-grilling or burning meats when grilling or on the barbecue. This triggers the formation of carcinogenic chemicals called heterocyclic amines (HCAs). If you like the smoky taste, marinate whatever

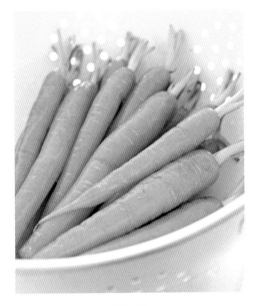

IS ORGANIC BETTER?

It does seem so, yes. Studies have shown that organic vegetables contain more antioxidants, vitamin C, iron and magnesium than intensively farmed ones – they also contain fewer heavy metals. If buying organic busts your budget, though, remember these tips:

- Scrub up: Washing produce does remove some pesticide residue.
- Up your portion sizes: While organic food may contain more nutrients, serving yourself a larger portion of conventional vegetables will make up the likely deficit for less cost.
- Buy smaller pieces: Studies have shown that the smaller the vegetable the more nutrients it contains – as produce grows it gets a higher portion of water, which dilutes its nutrient load.

you're cooking in a marinade containing rosemary for at least an hour prior to cooking – this cuts HCA formation by up to 80 per cent.

Set a treat limit Clear out that naughty cupboard (we all have one!) stuffed with crisps, salty snacks, cakes, biscuits and sweets, and buy them only sparingly – if they're not there you can't eat them.

Breakfast favourites

I HAVE OFTEN BEEN TOLD THAT BREAKFAST IS THE MOST IMPORTANT MEAL OF THE DAY – AND IT'S TRUE THAT BREAKFAST EATERS ARE MORE THAN FOUR TIMES LESS LIKELY TO BE OVERWEIGHT THAN THOSE WHO SKIP THE MEAL. THEY ALSO TAKE IN MORE NUTRIENTS THROUGHOUT THE DAY.

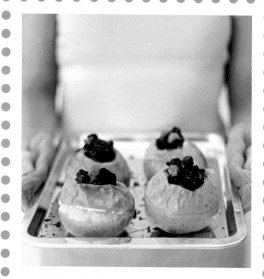

BAKED APPLE

This is super easy – leave it to cook while you get ready for the day

Serves 1

Core 1 large eating apple and score a line around the middle of the fruit. Stuff the cored centre with 25 g (1 oz) ready-to-eat dried fruit (cranberries, sultanas, apricots). Bake in a preheated oven, 200°C (400°F), Gas Mark 6, for 25 minutes. Serve with low-fat yogurt (optional).

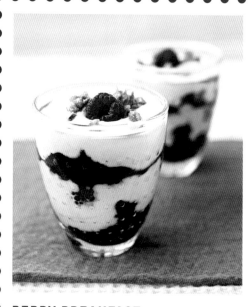

BERRY BREAKFAST

The luxurious mixture of rich yogurt and oats makes this breakfast deliciously creamy and satisfying

Serves 1

Put 75 ml (3 fl oz) low-fat Greek yogurt in a small bowl and fold in 2 teaspoons clear honey. Add 75 g (3 oz) raspberries and 1 tablespoon porridge oats and stir gently. Serve.

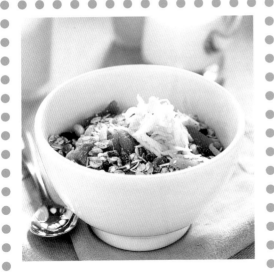

PUMPKIN SEED MUESLI
Make a huge batch of this, pop it in an airtight container and you're good to go

Makes 10 servings
Mix together 300 g (10 oz) rolled jumbo oats, 5 tablespoons sultanas or raisins, 5 tablespoons pumpkin seeds, 5 tablespoons chopped almonds and 150 g (5 oz) chopped ready-to-eat dried apricots and store. For each serving, add 2 tablespoons orange juice and 1 grated small apple, before topping with skimmed milk.

EGGS FLORENTINE
The healthy protein in this breakfast will keep you full until lunchtime

Serves 1
Heat 1 teaspoon olive oil in a nonstick frying pan and fry ½ finely chopped small onion for 3 minutes. Add 150 g (5 oz) defrosted frozen spinach leaves and a pinch of nutmeg and fry for a further 2–3 minutes. Stir in 1 tablespoon low-fat crème fraîche. Make a well in the centre of the spinach mixture. Crack in 1 egg and fry over a medium heat until the egg is cooked. Serve with 1 slice of wholemeal toast.

CREAMY MUSHROOM TOAST
This breakfast supplies you with one of your five daily fruit and vegetable portions

Serves 2
Toast 4 slices wholemeal bread in a toaster or under the grill. Meanwhile, heat 1 tablespoon avocado oil in a frying pan, add 1 tablespoon lime juice and fry 1 chopped small onion and 10 sliced mushrooms until soft. Stir in 1 tablespoon light soy sauce followed by 2 tablespoons ricotta cheese. Pour the mixture on top of the toast and serve.

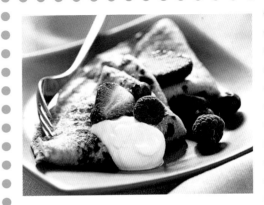

BUCKWHEAT PANCAKES
These pancakes are super-low GI

Serves 4
Sift 50 g (2 oz) wholemeal flour and 50 g (2 oz) buckwheat flour into a bowl, and add the grains left in the sieve. Beat together 1 egg and 300 ml (½ pint) skimmed milk then slowly add to the flour. Stir until a smooth batter forms. Leave to stand for 20 minutes, then stir again. Put 1 teaspoon of olive oil in a nonstick frying pan. When the pan is hot add 2 tablespoons of the pancake mixture and shake the pan to spread the mixture. Cook for 2 minutes, until the underside is lightly browned, turn the pancake over and cook the other side for a minute or so. Repeat. Serve topped with 1 piece chopped fresh fruit and 1–2 tablespoons low-fat yogurt.

Quick and easy lunches

WHETHER I'M AT HOME WITH MY FAMILY, OR WANT A HEALTHY OPTION TO TAKE INTO WORK, THERE ARE A HANDFUL SIMPLE LUNCH RECIPES THAT I FIND MYSELF RETURNING TO TIME AND AGAIN.

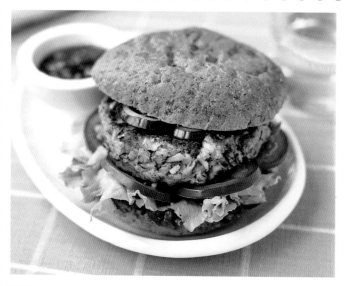

TURKEY BURGERS

The whole family will love these healthy burgers

Serves 4

In a bowl, mix together 250 g (8 oz) extra-lean minced turkey, 1 small grated onion, 2 small grated courgettes, 1 teaspoon soy sauce, 1 egg and 50 g (2 oz) each breadcrumbs and oatmeal. Cover and leave in the fridge for 30 minutes. Divide the mixture into 4 and shape the burgers with your hands. Grill for 6–7 minutes on each side until thoroughly cooked, then serve each burger in a granary roll stuffed with salad leaves, sliced tomatoes and onions.

MY MUM'S CHICKEN SOUP

This is a family favourite – it's really tasty, filling and comforting

Serves 6

Put 200–250 g (7–8 oz) chicken legs in a pan, cover with a little water and start cooking over a low heat. Chop 4–5 small carrots, 1 small turnip, 4 medium potatoes and 1 large leek. Slice 4 celery sticks, then add all the vegetables to the pan and simmer for 1 hour. Once the vegetables are soft, remove the chicken pieces and set aside. Pass the soup juice and vegetables through a strainer or blend in a food processor. Discard the chicken skin. Chop the meat into bite-sized pieces and return to the soup. Reheat the soup and garnish with chopped parsley to serve.

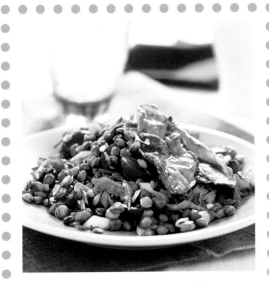

HERBY LENTIL SALAD WITH BACON

The lentils in this dish supply slow-release energy well into the afternoon

Serves 4

Fry 1 chopped garlic clove and 4 sliced spring onions for 2 minutes in a nonstick pan sprayed with a little oil. Add 2 x 400 g (13 oz) cans green lentils, drained and rinsed, 2 tablespoons balsamic vinegar, 3 tablespoon chopped herbs (such as parsley and oregano) and 125 g (4 oz) halved cherry tomatoes. Cook for 1 minute, then set aside. Grill 90 g (3¼ oz) back bacon rashers until crispy, then place on top of the salad.

MACKEREL PÂTÉ

Oily fish helps boost the health of your brain, skin and heart

Serves 1

Using a food processor, blend 100 g (3½ oz) peppered mackerel fillet, 25 g (1 oz) light cream cheese, 1 tablespoon light crème fraîche, 1 teaspoon creamed horseradish and 2 tablespoons mixed chopped herbs. Serve the pâté on rye crackers, with celery sticks.

LEMON TARRAGON CHICKEN SANDWICH ON RYE

Tasting as if it has come from the best sandwich shop, this is low calorie, low GI and low fat

Serves 4

In a bowl, mix together 3 tablespoons light crème fraîche, the grated rind and juice of 1 lemon, 1 tablespoon chopped tarragon, 8 sliced ready-to-eat dried apricots, 2 cooked boneless, skinless chicken breasts (about 150 g/5 oz each), shredded, and a large handful of rocket. Divide the mixture into quarters and use to sandwich 8 slices of rye bread.

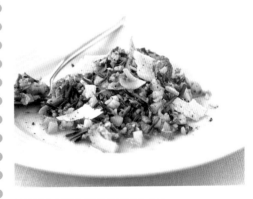

CRUNCHY RICE SALAD

Packed with B vitamins, this low-GI salad supplies slow-release energy

Serves 1

Cook 90 g (3 oz) each finely chopped broccoli, courgettes and peppers and 90 g (3 oz) finely sliced mushrooms in a large frying pan with a little water for 3–5 minutes, until softened. Reduce the heat to medium, then stir in 2 tablespoons pesto sauce, followed by 50 g (2 oz) each cooked brown and basmati rice and 25 g (1 oz) low-fat Parmesan. Remove the pan from the heat now if eating cold. If eating hot, cook for a further minute until the rice is warmed through.

Tasty dinners

I AM IN FAVOUR OF MAKING CHEAP EVENING
MEALS THAT ARE BURSTING WITH NUTRITION.
MY HUSBAND IS A FAR BETTER COOK THAN I
WILL EVER BE, AND I'M MORE THAN HAPPY
FOR HIM TO SHARE IN MAKING DISHES LIKE
THE ONES I'VE CHOSEN HERE!

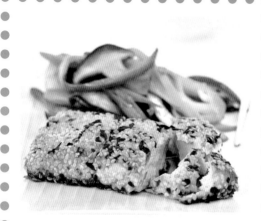

SESAME-CRUSTED SALMON
This speedy dish looks really special

Serves 4

Combine 4 tablespoons sesame seeds and
1 teaspoon dried chilli flakes on a plate, then
press 4 skinless salmon fillets (about 100 g/
3½ oz each) into this mixture, turning to coat
all sides. Heat 1 teaspoon olive oil in a nonstick
frying pan, add the salmon and cook over a
medium heat for 3–4 minutes on each side. Set
the salmon aside, keeping it warm. Thinly slice
2 red peppers, 2 carrots, 200 g (7 oz) shiitake
mushrooms, 2 pak choi and 4 spring onions.
Heat 1 teaspoon olive oil in the pan, add the
vegetables and quickly stir-fry for 3–4 minutes.
Drizzle 1 tablespoon soy sauce over the
vegetables then serve with the fish.

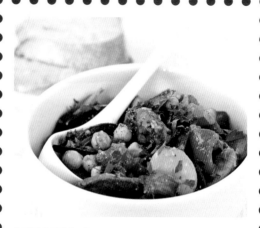

CHORIZO, CHICKPEA AND RED PEPPER STEW
*Cooking in one pot, this just needs a slice of
crusty bread to make it complete*

Serves 4

Cook 500 g (1 lb) new potatoes in boiling water
for 12–15 minutes, until tender. Drain, then
slice. Meanwhile, heat 1 teaspoon olive oil in a
large frying pan, add 2 chopped red onions and
2 cored, deseeded and chopped red peppers and
fry for 3–4 minutes. Add 100 g (3½ oz) thinly
sliced chorizo sausage and continue to fry for
2 minutes. Add the potato slices, 500 g (1 lb)
chopped plum tomatoes and 400 g (13 oz)
drained and rinsed canned chickpeas, bring to
the boil and simmer for 10 minutes. Serve with
crusty bread.

CHICKEN CURRY WITH BABY SPINACH

This curry is perfect for weekends: don't eat out, eat in, saving on both cash and calories

Serves 4

Chop in half 4 boneless, skinless chicken breasts (about 125 g/4 oz each) lengthways. Heat 1 tablespoon vegetable oil in a large nonstick saucepan. Add the chicken, 1 sliced onion, 2 chopped garlic cloves and 1 chopped green chilli and fry for 4–5 minutes. Stir in 4 lightly crushed cardamom pods and 1 teaspoon each of cumin seeds, dried chilli flakes, ground ginger and turmeric and fry for 1 more minute. Add 250 g (8 oz) baby spinach leaves to the pan, cover and cook gently until the leaves wilt, then stir in 300 g (10 oz) chopped tomatoes. Simmer for 15 minutes, removing the lid for the last 5 minutes. Stir in 150 ml (¼ pint) low-fat Greek yogurt and serve with basmati rice (optional).

CHEAT'S PAELLA

Purists may be horrified, but for a quick, easy supper this is hard to beat

Serves 4

Cut 2 boneless, skinless chicken breasts (about 125 g/4 oz each) into bite-sized pieces. Spray a large nonstick pan or wok with a little oil spray, add the chicken and fry until just about to brown. Remove the chicken from the pan and set aside. Core, deseed and chop 1 red and 1 green pepper, and chop 1 large onion and 1 garlic clove. Fry the peppers, onions and garlic for 3–4 minutes in the same frying pan. Add 400 g (13 oz) canned chopped tomatoes and return the chicken to the pan and simmer gently. Meanwhile, cook 250 g (8 oz) microwave golden rice as directed, then add this and 200 g (7 oz) mixed seafood to the pan. Sprinkle over the juice of 2 lemons and bubble on a high heat for 6–7 minutes until the seafood is cooked.

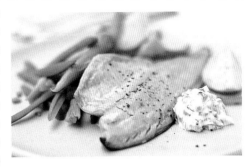

BAKED TROUT PARCELS WITH LOW-FAT TARTARE SAUCE

Healthy and simple. What more could you ask for in a dinner dish?

Serves 4

Prepare four trout parcels. Put a rainbow trout fillet (about 150 g/5 oz each) on an individual piece of foil and sprinkle the fillets with the rind and juice of 2 limes. Fold each piece of foil into a parcel, place on a baking sheet and bake in a preheated oven, 200°C (400°F), Gas Mark 6, for 12–15 minutes. Meanwhile make the tartare sauce. Combine in a small bowl 8 finely chopped cocktail gherkins, 4 teaspoons roughly chopped capers, 8 teaspoons low-fat crème fraîche, 4 sliced spring onions and 4 tablespoons chopped parsley and stir in the rind and juice of 2 limes. Remove the foil parcels from the oven, open, and carefully lift each trout on to a serving plate. Serve with the tartare sauce, new potatoes and vegetables.

BROCCOLI AND PINE NUT PASTA

This recipe is so easy, you wouldn't believe it could taste so good

Serves 4

Cut 600 g (1 lb 3 oz) broccoli into small florets. Cook 400 g (13 oz) pasta according to the packet instructions, adding the broccoli 5 minutes before the end of the cooking time. Drain the pasta and broccoli well, then add 50 g (2 oz) toasted pine nuts and 32 halved cherry tomatoes. Toss well and serve hot.

Delicious light suppers

SOMETIMES, AFTER A LONG DAY I DON'T WANT ANYTHING TOO HEAVY TO EAT COME THE EVENING MEAL. THESE LIGHT DISHES ARE SOME OF MY FAVOURITE SUPPER CHOICES.

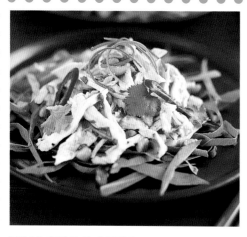

THAI-STYLE CHICKEN SALAD
This satisfies cravings for takeaway flavours

Serves 4
Mix 150 g (5 oz) shredded, ready-cooked chicken breast with 3 tablespoons coriander leaves. Make the dressing by putting 1 tablespoon groundnut oil, 1 tablespoon Thai fish sauce, the juice of 1 lime and 1 small orange, 1 crushed garlic clove and 3 tablespoons roughly chopped basil leaves in a screw-top jar, sealing the lid and shaking the jar to combine the ingredients. Pour the dressing over the chicken and stir to combine. Spoon the mixture on to 150 g (5 oz) shredded pak choi leaves and garnish with some red chilli slices.

CHEESE TORTILLAS
This is a perfectly delicious speedy meal

Serves 1
Make a salsa by combining 25 g (1 oz) ricotta cheese, ½ finely sliced red onion, 1 finely chopped tomato, ¼ finely chopped green chilli and 1 tablespoon chopped coriander in a bowl. Brush 2 small flour tortillas with a little oil, then cook very briefly on each side on a preheated hot griddle. Divide the salsa between the tortillas, spreading the mixture over one half of each. Fold over the second half of each tortilla and serve with a green salad.

ROSIE'S TUNA PASTA
This is one of my daughter Rosie's favourites and I always have the ingredients to hand

Serves 4
Cook 200 g (7 oz) pasta according to the packet instructions. Mix together 200 g (7 oz) canned tuna in oil and 1 tablespoon low-fat mayonnaise and add to the pasta. Stir in 2 tablespoons freshly grated Parmesan and season well with pepper. Serve with a green salad (optional).

SWEET POTATO AND GOATS' CHEESE FRITTATA

This summer favourite is perfect served simply, with a crisp green salad

Serves 4

Slice 500 g (1 lb) sweet potatoes. Place the sweet potato slices in a saucepan of boiling water and cook for 7–8 minutes until just tender, then drain. Heat 1 teaspoon olive oil in a nonstick frying pan, add 5 sliced spring onions and the sweet potato slices and fry for 2 minutes. Beat together 4 large eggs. Stir 2 tablespoons chopped coriander into the beaten eggs, season with plenty of pepper and pour into the pan. Cut 100 g (3½ oz) round goats' cheese with rind into 4 slices. Arrange the slices of goats' cheese on top of the egg and continue to cook for 3–4 minutes, until almost set. Place the pan under a high grill and cook for 2–3 minutes, until golden and bubbling. Serve hot.

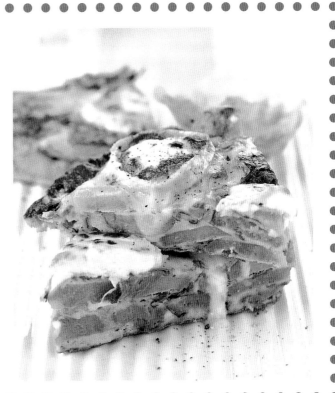

SMOKY BACON AND WHITE BEAN SOUP

If it's cold outside this quick, tasty soup will warm you up no end

Serves 4

Heat 1 teaspoon olive oil in a large saucepan, add 2 chopped rashers smoked bacon, 2 crushed garlic cloves, 1 chopped onion and fry for 3–4 minutes. Add 2–3 thyme sprigs and continue to fry for 1 minute, then add 800 g (26 oz) drained and rinsed canned cannellini beans and 900 ml (1½ pints) vegetable stock to the pan. Bring to the boil and simmer for 10 minutes. Transfer the soup to a blender or food processor and blend with 2 tablespoons chopped parsley and pepper to taste until the soup is smooth. Return the soup to the pan, heat through and serve with fresh wholegrain bread (optional).

WILD MUSHROOM OMELETTE

This mix of eggs, mushrooms and melted cheese makes for perfect comfort food

Serves 4

Chop 2 tablespoons parsley and grate 50 g (2 oz) Gruyère cheese and set them aside. Spray a nonstick frying pan with a little oil spray and fry 175 g (6 oz) trimmed and sliced wild mushrooms until soft. Remove from the pan. Beat together 8 large eggs. Spray the pan again, and add one-quarter of the beaten egg. Season well with pepper and stir with a wooden spoon, bringing the cooked egg to the centre of the pan and allowing the runny egg to flow to the edges. When there is only a little liquid egg left, sprinkle over a quarter of the mushrooms, parsley and cheese. Fold the omelette over and keep warm while you make 3 more omelettes in the same way.

Weight-watching

WHILE I TRY NEVER TO BEAT MYSELF UP
ABOUT THE SHAPE OF MY BODY, I KNOW THAT
BEING OVERWEIGHT DOES CARRY A HEAP OF
HEALTH RISKS. IT INCREASES YOUR RISK OF
HEART DISEASE BY UP TO 50 PER CENT AND
IS LINKED TO 12 DIFFERENT CANCERS.

WHAT IS A HEALTHY WEIGHT?

For most of us, the best way to determine this is to calculate something called our 'body mass index', which uses a mathematical equation to determine the health risk of an individual, and is a measure of obesity. While this doesn't work if you're an athlete packed head to toe with muscle, for the average woman it's a great way to see if you're at a healthy weight or not.

HOW TO CALCULATE YOUR BMI

The body mass index (BMI) is calculated as weight (kg/lb) divided by height (m/ft) squared ($BMI=kg/m2$).
For example, the BMI for someone who weighs 72 kg (159 lb), and is 1.64 m (5 ft 5 in) tall, is: 72 divided by 1.64 x 1.64 = 26.8. The readings of the BMI are:
• **BMI Less than 20:** Underweight
• **BMI 18.5–25:** Normal weight
• **BMI 25–30:** Overweight
• **BMI 30–40:** Obese

PILING ON THE POUNDS

Apart from a few people who gain weight for medical reasons, most of us put on pounds for one simple reason – we consume more calories than we use up each day. However, this simple fact can occur for hundreds of reasons. Say you serve yourself bigger portions without realizing, or you turn to comfort food at times of stress. Perhaps you gained weight during pregnancy and never lost it again, or have reduced the amount of activity you do. The good news is that virtually everyone can lose weight by eating less food and/or exercising more.

MIDDLE-AGED SPREAD

Many of us gain weight as we age – particularly around the tummy – which is bad news, because fat around your middle is particularly linked to a higher risk of health problems like heart disease. Many of us think this weight gain is a natural consequence of ageing, and that we can't do anything about it, but medical experts say this isn't strictly true. Although it's correct that the average woman burns 150 calories fewer a day past the age of 35, only 50 of these calories are lost owing to biological reasons (for example, the amount of calorie-burning muscle we have in our body declines). The remaining 100 calories are lost simply because we move less as we get older. Adding a 30-minute walk a day (or 15 minutes of intense exercise) will rebalance the calories in, calories out deficit again, while helping to build muscle and better bone health.

SLIMMING MIRACLES

These days would-be dieters are bombarded with promises of miracle cures from those promoting

CALCULATE YOUR BMI

The dotted line represents the BMI of someone who is 1.7 m (5 ft 7 in) tall and weighs 82 kg (13 stone), giving a BMI reading in the top end of the overweight category.

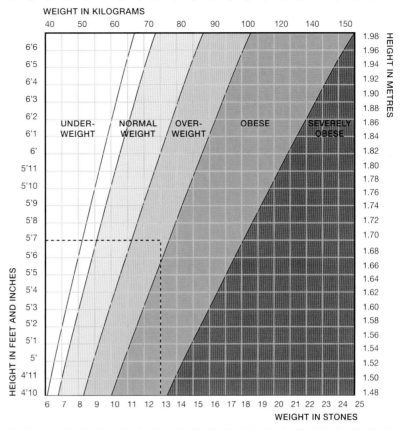

fad diets, cosmetic surgery or special pills. Here's the lowdown:

The fad diet Most celebrity-led, fad diets are impossible to stick to. They see you cutting calories to unsustainable low levels, dumping entire food groups or substituting real food for shakes or soups that you can't live on forever.

The gastric band While a gastric band – literally a band placed around the stomach to reduce the amount of food it can hold – does lead to massive weight loss, it involves major surgery and can lead to further problems, such as stomach ulcers and acid reflux. There is also a risk of band slippage, which might see a need for more surgery within 3–4 years.

Tummy tucks Going under the knife is a huge commitment with real health risks. Furthermore,

about 10 per cent of any cosmetic surgery needs redoing. Anyone considering surgical measures should investigate things very thoroughly, and make absolutely sure the doctor is qualified to do the operation.

Liposuction While liposuction removes subcutaneous fat from one area of your body (using suction), if you gain weight afterwards, the fat will go back on elsewhere and this can leave you with some very odd lumps and bumps, which will look very odd.

Slimming pills Claiming to speed up metabolism or reduce appetite, many of these offer almost effortless-sounding weight loss. However, none of them teach you how to eat properly, and as soon as you come off the pills, you'll fall back into your normal eating habits.

The real woman's weight-loss plan

WELCOME TO MY WEIGHT-LOSS PLAN. FOLLOW THE WEEKLY PLANS (SEE PAGES 38–49) AND YOU COULD LOSE UP TO A STONE OVER THE NEXT SIX WEEKS.

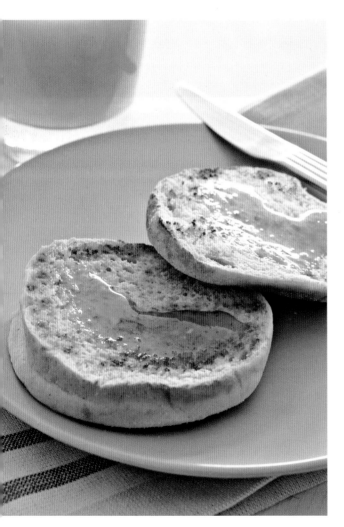

CHANGING YOUR HABITS

Please note that I'm not calling this a diet. I really believe that we have to get out of the mindset of being 'on' a diet because, inevitably, you will find yourself having come 'off' the diet and reverting to your old ways. If you want to drop a dress size or lose a stone – and have it stay off – then you have to tell yourself that the changes you're making in your eating and exercise habits (eating plenty of fruit and vegetables, choosing wholegrain carbohydrates, reducing fat levels by cutting obvious fat from meat and choosing low-fat versions of dairy and other products) are ones that you'll adopt in the longer term.

This isn't a crash, six-week plan. Of course, it will work as such in the short term, but your focus should be on the future, when you will break free of the tyranny of diets and be able to eat the food you enjoy without feeling guilty. That's what this plan aims to do – it doesn't ban any foods, but offers the healthiest versions of all the food groups, while giving you regular treats. It is not extremely low in calories either, which means you won't be derailed by hunger pangs. It's also easy to fit around work and home, as it does not rely on you having to cook complicated lunchtime meals, and is suitable for the whole family. But before you get started there's one more thing I'm going to suggest.

KEEPING A FOOD DIARY

Many of us have a very strange relationship with food, and until each of us understands why we choose the foods we eat, we will struggle to achieve that balance that allows us to eat the things we love without putting on weight. This is why, even if you're following an organized eating plan, keeping a food diary can help you. Instead of simply writing down everything you eat, ask yourself questions about the food you've consumed. Did the meal satisfy you? What did you enjoy most about it?

If certain cravings hit, use your food diary to find out why. Do you crave sweet food around 11 am or want potato crisps late at night? Ask yourself why that should be? I always used to have a cup of tea while watching TV at around 8 pm. This would have been fine, had I not thought that there was something unnatural about a cup of tea without a chocolate biscuit, and I found it hard to stick at just one once the packet was open. I managed to break this habit of mindless overeating by swapping regular tea for a peppermint or chamomile version. You don't add milk or sugar to these teas and they just don't 'go' with cakes or biscuits. You can use your diary to try to spot and break your 'bad' habits in the same way. If you manage this, the weight loss you achieve is more likely to stay gone for good.

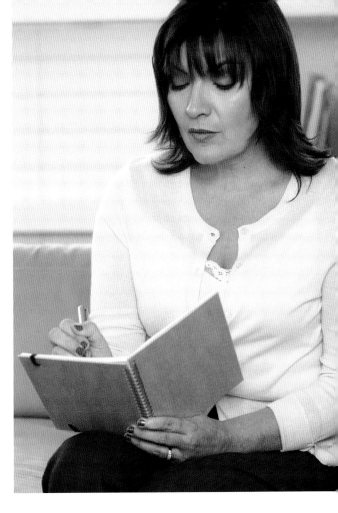

HOW TO USE MY WEIGHT-LOSS PLAN

Simply follow the plan as directed, but remember that you're trying to make this something you can follow for life. If you don't like a particular food in any meal, feel free to swap it for something similar that you do like. For example, change chicken to fish, green beans to broccoli, oranges to apples and so on. Also, while the plan offers you plenty of variety, you can repeat meals from other days if that suits your budget,

IF YOU WANT TO LOSE A STONE – AND HAVE IT STAY OFF – THEN YOU NEED TO ADOPT THESE LIFESTYLE CHANGES FOR THE LONG TERM

shopping style or taste buds better. Bear in mind that you should try not to eat the same thing more than three times a week, as this limits the variety of nutrients you'll take in. You can also swap any meal for any of the recipe suggestions on pages 26–33 so long as you replace like with like (a lunch with a lunch, for example). Just make sure that together the meals and snacks provide you with your five portions (at least) of fruit and vegetables a day. I've not included drinks on every page, but ideally you should aim for eight glasses of low- or no-calorie fluid a day – that means water, diet soft drinks, tea or herbal tea.

Week one

DAY ONE

BREAKFAST 40 g (1½ oz) porridge oats made up as directed, with 150 ml (¼ pint) skimmed milk. Add 1 chopped apple and 1 tablespoon sultanas.

LUNCH 400 g (13 oz) can of any bean- or lentil-based soup with a small wholemeal pitta filled with 1 boiled egg, 1 teaspoon low-fat salad dressing and salad.

DINNER 125 g (4 oz) chicken breast, stir-fried with Chinese cabbage, carrots and green pepper in a little sesame oil, chilli and soy sauce. Serve with 50 g (2 oz) egg noodles (dry weight).

SNACKS/TREATS Choose any two from: 125 g (4 oz) low-fat yogurt; 1 piece of fruit (orange, apple); 4 squares of any dark chocolate.

DAY TWO

BREAKFAST 1 boiled egg, served with 2 slices of granary toast and yeast-extract spread and 1 piece of fruit.

LUNCH 75 g (3 oz) basmati rice (dry weight), boiled then mixed with 125 g (4 oz) canned salmon and some chopped tomato. Serve with sliced cucumber.

DINNER 1 low-fat quarter-pounder or veggie burger, grilled, topped with 200 g (7 oz) canned ratatouille and 200 g (7 oz) mashed potato.

SNACKS/TREATS Choose any two from: 200 g (7 oz) fruit cocktail in natural juice; 3 chocolate finger biscuits; 1 tablespoon hummus with 5 cucumber sticks.

DAY THREE

BREAKFAST 40 g (1½ oz) any low-sugar cereal, served with 200 ml (7 fl oz) skimmed milk and 1 banana.

LUNCH 250 g (8 oz) baked potato, topped with 3 tablespoons low-fat coleslaw and 25 g (1 oz) low-fat Cheddar cheese or 75 g (3 oz) canned tuna.

DINNER 125 g (4 oz) salmon or trout fillet, grilled and served with 4–5 new potatoes, a dab of mayonnaise or horseradish and unlimited green beans and carrots.

SNACKS/TREATS Choose any two from: 1 slice of watermelon; 1 crumpet topped with low-sugar jam; 1 sachet of low-calorie hot chocolate made with skimmed milk.

DAY FOUR

BREAKFAST 1 wholewheat tortilla filled with 1 chopped peach, pear or apple and 1 handful of strawberries, served with 125 g (4 oz) low-fat yogurt.

LUNCH 3 slices of lean ham (or 1 boiled egg) and 200 g (7 oz) supermarket bean salad, served with spinach and carrot salad.

DINNER 50 g (2 oz) pasta spirals (dry weight), boiled then topped with a sauce made from 150 g (5 oz) canned tuna, onion and courgettes, simmered in 150 g (5 oz) canned tomatoes, mixed herbs and garlic for 15–20 minutes.

SNACKS/TREATS Choose any two from: 1 chocolate digestive biscuit; 25 g (1 oz) low-fat cheese with 2–3 pickled onions; a 125 ml (4 fl oz) glass of wine.

DAY FIVE

BREAKFAST 1 piece of toast topped with 200 g (7 oz) low-sugar baked beans, served with 2 pieces of fruit.

LUNCH 6-piece sushi pack from any supermarket, served with a small side salad of chopped cabbage and apple.

DINNER Shepherd's pie made from 125 g (4 oz) lean mince, browned then drained. Add 1 chopped carrot, 2 tablespoons sweetcorn and 100 ml (4 fl oz) gravy. Simmer until the carrot is cooked, then reduce so that all the liquid disappears. Top with 200 g (7 oz) mashed potato, grill until brown and serve with unlimited broccoli.

SNACKS/TREATS Choose any two from: 100 g (3½ oz) low-fat rice pudding; 200 g (7 oz) canned pears or peaches; 1 small handful of almonds.

DAY SIX

BREAKFAST Small reduced-fat croissant, served with a little low-sugar jam and 2 pieces of fruit.

LUNCH 125 g (4 oz) slice of any low-fat quiche, served with 2 tablespoons low-fat coleslaw and unlimited salad.

DINNER Roast 125 g (4 oz) chicken breast for 15–20 minutes in a preheated oven, 200°C (400°F), Gas Mark 6. Slice in half, add 1 teaspoon pesto, 1 slice ham and 3 slices red pepper. Return to the oven for 5 minutes. Serve with a green salad and 4–5 new potatoes.

SNACKS/TREATS Choose any two from: ½ apple dipped in 1 teaspoon peanut butter; 2 shortbread biscuits; 1 piece of toast with a little yeast-extract spread.

DAY SEVEN

BREAKFAST 2 slices of back bacon (fat removed) and 1 tomato, grilled, with 1 piece of toast.

LUNCH 200 g (7 oz) canned vegetable chilli. Serve with green salad and the wedges of 1 large sweet potato, sprayed lightly with an oil spray and baked in a preheated oven, 200°C (400°F), Gas Mark 6, for 20–25 minutes.

DINNER 125 g (4 oz) white fish fillet, pan-fried with a little Cajun spice, with 50 g (2 oz) brown rice (dry weight) and unlimited broccoli.

SNACKS/TREATS Choose any two from: 1 pack of low-fat potato crisps; 1 large banana; 1 pot of low-fat chocolate mousse.

Week two

DAY ONE

BREAKFAST 2 eggs, scrambled with a little skimmed milk, in a wholewheat tortilla with 1 tablespoon salsa. Serve with 1 orange.

LUNCH 200 g (7 oz) any low-fat pasta salad, served with a large green salad and 125 g (4 oz) sliced chicken or 50 g (2 oz) roasted red peppers (from the deli) and 25 g (1 oz) feta cheese.

DINNER 125 g (4 oz) gammon steak, grilled, with 200 g (7 oz) butter beans, mashed with a little low-fat crème fraîche, and unlimited broccoli.

SNACKS/TREATS Choose any two from: 1 cereal bar (under 100 calories); ½ banana and 3 Brazil nuts; 25 g (1 oz) Brie with ½ peach.

DAY TWO

BREAKFAST 5 chopped dried apricots and 1 handful of almonds mixed into 125 g (4 oz) low-fat yogurt.

LUNCH ½ carton of any vegetable soup, served with 2–3 oatcakes topped with ½ avocado, mashed.

DINNER 75 g (3 oz) any pasta (dry weight), boiled and topped with 1 tablespoon pesto sauce and a mix of grilled courgettes and red/yellow pepper strips.

SNACKS/TREATS Choose any two from: ½ hot cross bun; 4–5 dried apple chips; 200 g (7 oz) canned strawberries in natural juice.

DAY THREE

BREAKFAST 1 slice of granary toast topped with 1 teaspoon peanut butter and 1 mashed banana, with 200 ml (7 fl oz) skimmed milk or a milky coffee on the side.

LUNCH Tuna niçoise-style salad, made from unlimited green beans, tomato, onion and 4 black olives mixed with 125 g (4 oz) tuna and 1 boiled egg. Serve with 1 small slice of crusty bread.

DINNER Top 1 aubergine, halved and roasted until soft in the oven, with a little olive oil, with 50 g (2 oz) feta cheese and 25 g (1 oz) pine nuts and serve with 50 g (2 oz) basmati rice (dry weight).

SNACKS/TREATS Choose any two from: 75 g (3 oz) low-fat cottage cheese with pineapple; ½ mango, fresh or grilled; 25 g (1 oz) snack pack of raisins.

DAY FOUR

BREAKFAST 40 g (1½ oz) porridge oats or 40 g (1½ oz) any low-sugar cereal, with 150 ml (¼ pint) skimmed milk, 1 chopped apple or pear and 1 tablespoon sultanas.

LUNCH Any ready-made supermarket sandwich (under 300 calories), with 1 low-fat yogurt and 1 piece of fruit.

DINNER 150 g (5 oz) trout, grilled, with 200 g (7 oz) mashed sweet potato and unlimited green beans or mangetout.

SNACKS/TREATS Choose any two from: 1 low-fat choc ice; 1 baked apple (see recipe on page 26); 2 slices of lean ham, each wrapped round 1 small slice of avocado.

DAY FIVE

BREAKFAST 1 ready-made cereal bar with 125 g (4 oz) low-fat yogurt and any 2 pieces of fruit.

LUNCH 125 g (4 oz) fresh prawns and ½ chopped avocado, mixed with 1 tablespoon salsa and served on a bed of lettuce and cucumber.

DINNER 1 low-fat sausage, grilled, with a 250 g (8 oz) baked potato and 3 tablespoons low-fat coleslaw.

SNACKS/TREATS Choose any two from: 2 rye crackers topped with 25 g (1 oz) low-fat cream cheese and sliced strawberries; ½ pear dipped into 1 teaspoon peanut butter; 1 handful of any jelly sweets.

DAY SIX

BREAKFAST French toast, made from 1 slice of bread soaked in a mix of 1 egg and a little skimmed milk, then fried in a little oil spray, served with 1 sliced tomato or 2 handfuls of berries.

LUNCH Caesar-style salad made from iceberg lettuce tossed in low-fat Caesar dressing with 1–2 sliced radishes, 125 g (4 oz) grilled chicken and 1 boiled egg.

DINNER 125 g (4 oz) chicken tikka fillets (from the supermarket) or 1 Quorn™ fillet, served with a 200 g (7 oz) selection of mixed vegetables (carrot, cauliflower, broccoli) cooked with 3 tablespoons ready-made curry sauce.

SNACKS/TREATS Choose any two from: 75 g (3 oz) low-fat vanilla ice cream; 2 Bourbon biscuits; 1 unit of spirits with a diet mixer.

DAY SEVEN

BREAKFAST 2 slices of raisin toast, spread with a little low-fat spread and served with 1 sliced banana.

LUNCH 125 g (4 oz) any roast meat, 3 small roast potatoes, unlimited vegetables and 1 tablespoon gravy.

DINNER 125 g (4 oz) canned salmon with 200 g (7 oz) ready-made potato salad (or 4–5 new potatoes, cooked, sliced and mixed with a little low-fat dressing) and unlimited green salad.

SNACKS/TREATS Choose any two from: 1 mini chocolate Swiss roll; 200 ml (7 fl oz) skimmed milk; 3 walnuts.

Week three

DAY ONE

BREAKFAST 40 g (1½ oz) any low-sugar cereal, served with 150 ml (¼ pint) skimmed milk, 1 tablespoon sultanas or 5 chopped dried apricots and ½ banana, chopped.

LUNCH 200 g (7 oz) canned tuna, mackerel, salmon or sardines mixed with a little low-fat mayonnaise and served with crudités of carrot, celery, cucumber and cherry tomatoes.

DINNER 1 fillet of cod in breadcrumbs, with 200 g (7 oz) oven chips or wedges and 2 grilled tomatoes.

SNACKS/TREATS Choose any two from: 1 low-fat yogurt drink; 50 g (2 oz) dried banana chips; 1 English muffin topped with a little honey.

DAY TWO

BREAKFAST 2 wholewheat tortillas, filled with 125 g (4 oz) low-fat cottage cheese and pineapple and served with 3 handfuls of berries.

LUNCH 250 g (8 oz) baked potato, topped with 200 g (7 oz) baked beans and served with 1 piece of fruit.

DINNER Stir-fry 125 g (4 oz) firm tofu and 25 g (1 oz) cashew nuts with unlimited mushrooms and bean sprouts in 2 teaspoons sesame oil, a little chilli and some soy sauce. Serve with 50 g (2 oz) brown rice (dry weight).

SNACKS/TREATS Choose any two from: 1 biscotti and a small cappuccino; 3 kiwifruit; 2 celery sticks dipped in 1 teaspoon peanut butter.

DAY THREE

BREAKFAST 1 apple and 1 pear, sliced, dipped into 2 teaspoons peanut butter and served with 125 g (4 oz) low-fat yogurt.

LUNCH Sandwich made from 2 slices of granary or rye bread, spread with 25 g (1 oz) low-fat soft cheese and 50 g (2 oz) smoked salmon and served with slices of cucumber or 1 pickled gherkin.

DINNER Vegetarian lasagne, made from layering a mix of chopped courgettes, aubergine and red pepper simmered in 125 g (4 oz) ready-made tomato pasta sauce and 4 tablespoons ready-made cheese sauce between 4 sheets of lasagne pasta prepared as directed on the packet. Cook in a preheated oven, 200°C (400°F), Gas Mark 6, for 20 minutes, then serve with green beans.

SNACKS/TREATS Choose any two from: 1 small handful of dried roasted peanuts; 4 strawberries dipped in 1 teaspoon low-fat chocolate spread; 2 oatcakes topped with 1 teaspoon lemon curd.

DAY FOUR

BREAKFAST 2 slices of wholegrain toast, topped with 1 mashed banana, with 200 ml (7 fl oz) skimmed milk or a milky coffee on the side.

LUNCH 200 g (7 oz) any low-fat supermarket rice, pasta or potato salad, served with 200 g (7 oz) canned salmon and one-quarter bag of any supermarket leaf salad.

DINNER 125 g (4 oz) lean steak (or a Quorn™/salmon fillet), grilled or pan-fried with oil spray and served with 2 tablespoons low-fat coleslaw, 1 small corn on the cob and 3 new potatoes.

SNACKS/TREATS Choose any two from: ½ pear served with 1 mini-Edam cheese; 2 fig roll biscuits; 3 large, flavoured rice cakes.

DAY FIVE

BREAKFAST 1 English muffin topped with 1 teaspoon low-fat jam or honey, with 200 ml (7 fl oz) fruit juice on the side.

LUNCH Ploughman-style lunch made from 50 g (2 oz) any low-fat cheese, 3 pickled onions, 2 celery sticks, 1 carrot cut into sticks, a little salsa and 2 rye crackers.

DINNER 125 g (4 oz) pork chop (fat removed), served with 3 small roast potatoes, 1 teaspoon apple sauce and unlimited peas.

SNACKS/TREATS Choose any two from: 1 Melba toast topped with 25 g (1 oz) soft cheese; 1 meringue nest filled with 1 tablespoon low-fat yogurt and 1 handful of berries; 5 Brazil nuts.

DAY SIX

BREAKFAST Smoothie made from 200 ml (7 oz) skimmed milk, 1 banana and 2–3 handfuls of berries, served with 1 slice of toast or 3 rice cakes.

LUNCH Salmon cakes. Boil, grate and cool 150 g (5 oz) potatoes, mix with 25 g (1 oz) low-fat Cheddar and 50 g (2 oz) canned salmon, form into a patty and pan-fry with a little oil spray. Serve with a large green salad or boiled green beans.

DINNER 4 tablespoons of any chicken or fish dish from the Chinese or Indian takeaway, with 4 tablespoons plain boiled rice and 3 tablespoons of any vegetable dish.

SNACKS/TREATS Choose any two from: 1 small ice lolly; 2 custard cream biscuits; 5 prunes – dried or canned in natural juice.

DAY SEVEN

BREAKFAST 2 slices of toast, each topped with 25 g (1 oz) low-fat grated Cheddar and grilled. Serve with 2 sliced tomatoes.

LUNCH Omelette made from 2 eggs and filled with your choice of red peppers, courgette, mushrooms and onion, served with 200 g (7 oz) baked beans or a green salad.

DINNER 125 g (4 oz) calamari rings in batter, grilled, with 50 g (2 oz) brown rice (dry weight) and a little sweet chilli sauce. Serve with stir-fried spinach or Chinese cabbage.

SNACKS/TREATS Choose any two from: 25 g (1 oz) slice of angel cake; 1 tablespoon salsa served with 10 corn chips; 1 small pot of fruit purée.

Week four

BREAKFAST 40 g (1½ oz) Bircher-style muesli (made as directed with skimmed milk), topped with 1 sliced banana.

LUNCH 2 slices of toast topped with 200 g (7 oz) baked beans and sausages and served with 1 piece of fruit.

DINNER 350 g (11½ oz) low-fat cauliflower cheese, with 200 g (7 oz) canned ratatouille.

SNACKS/TREATS Choose any two from: 125 g (4 oz) low-fat Greek yogurt with a dab of honey; 300 ml (½ pint) lager; 1 large rice cake spread with 1 teaspoon chocolate spread.

BREAKFAST 25 g (1 oz) any low-fat cheese, 2 slices of ham, 1 sliced tomato and 1 piece of rye bread.

LUNCH 250 g (8 oz) baked potato topped with 125 g (4 oz) sardines in tomato sauce, with a green salad.

DINNER 125 g (4 oz) lamb chop served with ½ large roasted parsnip and 200 g (7 oz) mushy peas.

SNACKS/TREATS Choose any two from: 1 lemon and raisin pancake (from the supermarket); 1 tablespoon of any dip served with 1 handful of baby carrots; ½ small blueberry muffin.

BREAKFAST 2 slices of wholegrain toast topped with 200 g (7 oz) canned tomatoes and 1 slice of ham or grilled back bacon.

LUNCH Salad of lettuce, cucumber and celery, tossed in a little low-fat ranch dressing and topped with 1 sliced apple, 3 walnuts and 125 g (4 oz) prawns.

DINNER 125 g (4 oz) pan-fried lamb's liver, with fried onions, 200 g (7 oz) mashed sweet potatoes and unlimited broccoli.

SNACKS/TREATS Choose any two from: 25 g (1 oz) low-fat Cheddar on 1 cracker; 125 g (4 oz) rhubarb stewed until soft with a little sugar; 150 ml (5 oz) yogurt drink.

DAY FOUR

BREAKFAST 1 scrambled egg, with 200 g (7 oz) low-sugar baked beans.

LUNCH ½ carton of any fresh soup with 1 large slice of ciabatta bread topped with a salsa-style mix of chopped tomato and onion.

DINNER Chilli con carne, made with 75 g (3 oz) lean mince and ⅓ jar of ready-made chilli sauce, served with 50 g (2 oz) basmati rice (dry weight) and a side of wilted spinach.

SNACKS/TREATS Choose any two from: 2.5 cm (1 inch) slice of fruit loaf; 2 rye crackers topped with mashed banana; 3 satsumas/fresh apricots.

DAY FIVE

BREAKFAST 40 g (1½ oz) any low-sugar cereal, served with 200 ml (7 fl oz) skimmed milk, 1 sliced apple and 5 dried apricots.

LUNCH Club sandwich made from 3 slices of granary bread, 1 slice of ham, 1 slice of chicken, 1 sliced boiled egg and 1 sliced tomato, served with cucumber and carrot sticks.

DINNER 125 g (4 oz) fresh tuna steak, grilled or pan-fried, with 200 g (7 oz) mashed potato and unlimited broccoli.

SNACKS/TREATS Choose any two from: 25 g (1 oz) any cheese with 1 teaspoon chutney; 1 Scotch pancake topped with 1 squirt of aerosol cream and some fresh strawberries; 30 ml (1¼ fl oz) creamy liqueur.

DAY SIX

BREAKFAST Salmon cakes, with unlimited grilled tomatoes and mushrooms.

LUNCH 1 quarter-pounder burger, grilled well and served in a wholegrain bun with pan-fried onions, green salad and 1 teaspoon of avocado.

DINNER 6 scallops lightly pan-fried, with 50 g (2 oz) brown rice (dry weight), roasted courgette and red and yellow peppers.

SNACKS/TREATS Choose any two from: 10 black or green olives with 25 g (1 oz) feta cheese; 1 pear poached in a little fruit juice; 30 g (1¼ oz) fruit or nut bar.

DAY SEVEN

BREAKFAST 1 sweet waffle topped with 3 handfuls of any berry and 125 g (4 oz) low-fat yogurt.

LUNCH 125 g (4 oz) lean roast beef served with 1 small individual Yorkshire pudding, unlimited vegetables and 1 tablespoon gravy.

DINNER 400 g (13 oz) can of any soup, with 2 slices of granary toast topped with 25 g (1 oz) grated cheese, grilled well.

SNACKS/TREATS Choose any two from: 2 cheese straws dipped into 1 tablespoon salsa; protein shake made from 200 ml (7 fl oz) skimmed milk and a scoop of protein powder; 3 handfuls of any berry.

Week five

DAY ONE

BREAKFAST ½ blueberry bagel topped with 25 g (1 oz) low-fat cream cheese, served with 2 slices canned or fresh pineapple and 1 orange.

LUNCH Salad of rocket tossed in a little balsamic vinegar, topped with 125 g (4 oz) prawns, 25 g (1 oz) fresh Parmesan and some sliced cherry tomatoes.

DINNER 125 g (4 oz) lean steak (or Quorn™ fillet), grilled, with ½ roasted aubergine and 3 roast potatoes.

SNACKS/TREATS Choose any two from: 1 inch (2.5 cm) slice of malt loaf; 2 cheese triangles with cucumber slices; 1 fondant fancy cake.

DAY TWO

BREAKFAST 40 g (1½ oz) porridge oats made with water, topped with 1 chopped pear, 3 chopped dried apricots and 125 g (4 oz) low-fat yogurt.

LUNCH 2 pieces of toast topped with 150 g (5 oz) sardines in tomato sauce, followed by 1 pot of yogurt and 1 piece of fruit.

DINNER 125 g (4 oz) chicken breast, basted with a little harissa sauce and grilled, served with 50 g (2 oz) couscous (dry weight) and 3 tablespoons low-fat coleslaw.

SNACKS/TREATS Choose any two from: 100-calorie chocolate bar; 3 crabsticks with 1 tablespoon low-fat coleslaw; 1 small handful of yogurt-covered raisins.

DAY THREE

BREAKFAST 2 slices of raisin toast, topped with a little low-fat spread and served with 1 piece of fruit and 200 ml (7 fl oz) skimmed milk or a milky coffee on the side.

LUNCH 200 g (7 oz) any supermarket ready-made pasta, rice or bean salad, served with 125 g (4 oz) tuna (in brine) and some slices of beetroot.

DINNER 1 sachet of cod in butter, parsley or other sauce, served with 200 g (7 oz) oven chips and unlimited broccoli.

SNACKS/TREATS Choose any two from: 2 small chocolate-chip biscuits; fruit salad made from 2 different chopped fruits and 1 teaspoon single cream; baby carrots dipped into 1 tablespoon tzatziki.

DAY FOUR

BREAKFAST Smoothie made from 125 g (4 oz) low-fat yogurt, 100 ml (3½ fl oz) skimmed milk and 3 handfuls of any berry, served with 3 flavoured rice cakes.

LUNCH Any supermarket sandwich (under 300 calories), served with carrot sticks and red pepper slices dipped into 1 tablespoon salsa or hummus.

DINNER 125 g (4 oz) lamb chop or 50 g (2 oz) haloumi cheese, grilled well, served with 50 g (2 oz) brown rice (dry weight) and unlimited roasted red pepper, aubergine and courgette, topped with 1 tablespoon tzatziki.

SNACKS/TREATS Choose any two from: 25 g (1 oz) low-fat pâté with celery sticks; 2-finger chocolate-covered wafer bar; 125 g (4 oz) soya yogurt.

DAY FIVE

BREAKFAST 50 g (2 oz) fruit scone topped with 1 teaspoon low-sugar jam and 1 sliced pear or apple.

LUNCH Tortilla wrap spread with a little salsa and filled with 75 g (3 oz) prawns or tuna and 1 tablespoon low-fat coleslaw, served with a small pack of low-fat potato crisps.

DINNER 50 g (2 oz) pasta (dry weight), boiled and topped with a bolognaise sauce made from 75 g (3 oz) lean beef mince (or vegetarian mince alternative), unlimited mushrooms and ⅛ jar of ready-made tomato pasta sauce.

SNACKS/TREATS Choose any two from: 1 brandy snap filled with chopped canned peaches and topped with 1 tablespoon low-fat Greek yogurt; 1 handful of unsalted pretzels; 3 slices canned pineapple.

DAY SIX

BREAKFAST 1 small wholemeal roll, spread with a little ketchup or brown sauce and filled with 2 slices of grilled back bacon or 1 low-fat meat or vegetarian sausage and sliced tomatoes. Serve with 200 ml (7 fl oz) fruit juice.

LUNCH Omelette made from 2 eggs, filled with 25 g (1 oz) grated cheese and unlimited mushrooms, served with 2 tablespoons low-fat coleslaw and some beetroot slices.

DINNER 2 slices of any thin-crust takeaway pizza, served with a small green salad.

SNACKS/TREATS Choose any two from: 2 Jaffa cakes, 5 dried apricots; 1 digestive biscuit spread with a little low-fat spread.

DAY SEVEN

BREAKFAST 2 lemon and raisin pancakes, served with 125 g (4 oz) low-fat yogurt mixed with 3 handfuls of any berry.

LUNCH 125 g (4 oz) roast beef (or 2 small roast potatoes for a meat-free option), served with 300 g (10 oz) low-fat cauliflower cheese and unlimited cabbage or broccoli.

DINNER 1 large field mushroom, grilled and topped with a mix of chopped tomato and 25 g (1 oz) feta cheese, served with a large green salad.

SNACKS/TREATS Choose any two from: 1 boiled egg, mashed and served with celery sticks; 25 g (1 oz) any cereal with a splash of milk; 15 g (½ oz) chocolate buttons.

Week six

DAY ONE

BREAKFAST 200 g (7 oz) any fruit canned in natural juice, served with 125 g (4 oz) low-fat fromage frais and 1 handful of almonds or pumpkin seeds.

LUNCH 250 g (8 oz) baked potato, topped with 200 g (7 oz) of baked beans and 25 g (1 oz) grated cheese.

DINNER Stir-fry 125 g (4 oz) lean pork (or tofu) with ½ apple, ½ red pepper and ½ onion (all chopped), a little fresh root ginger and a splash of soy sauce. Serve with 50 g (2 oz) brown rice (dry weight).

SNACKS/TREATS Choose any two from: 1 large water biscuit topped with 1 teaspoon of pesto sauce and a thin slice of buffalo mozzarella; 25 g (1 oz) slice of carrot cake; 2 handfuls of cherries.

DAY TWO

BREAKFAST 2 slices of toast, served with ½ avocado, mashed, and sliced tomatoes.

LUNCH Small pack of vegetarian sushi and 1 sachet of miso soup, followed by 1 orange.

DINNER 125 g (4 oz) lean steak, pan-fried, or 1 Quorn™ steak, served with a purée of 150 g (5 oz) sweet potato and 50 g (2 oz) cauliflower, and unlimited mangetout.

SNACKS/TREATS Choose any two from: 3 squares of fudge; 3 fresh dates; 2 slices of roast beef, spread with mustard and wrapped around cucumber sticks.

DAY THREE

BREAKFAST 2 wholegrain cereal biscuits, topped with 150 ml (¼ pint) skimmed milk and 1 sliced pear, peach or apple.

LUNCH 1 small pitta, filled with 25 g (1 oz) soft cheese such as Brie and slices of red and yellow pepper, served with 3 tablespoons of low-fat coleslaw.

DINNER Grilled kebabs made from 125 g (4 oz) firm white fish (such as monkfish) alternated with pieces of pineapple, red pepper and courgette.

SNACKS/TREATS Choose any two from: 1 small handful of cashew nuts; 125 ml (4 fl oz) glass of champagne; 1 slice of toast topped with 1 slice of processed cheese.

DAY FOUR

BREAKFAST Large slice of watermelon, served with 1 slice of toast and 100 g (3½ oz) low-fat cottage cheese.

LUNCH Greek-style salad, made from chopped tomato, cucumber and onion, topped with 5 black olives and 50 g (2 oz) low-fat feta.

DINNER 125 g (4 oz) salmon steak, grilled, served with 4 tablespoons low-fat potato salad and 5 spears of asparagus.

SNACKS/TREATS Choose any two from: 2 pieces of sushi; 200 ml (7 fl oz) of any soup; 3 mini chocolate eggs.

DAY FIVE

BREAKFAST 40 g (1½ oz) porridge oats made with water and topped with 1 teaspoon cinnamon and 125 g (4 oz) low-fat yogurt.

LUNCH 2 slices of toast, topped with 200 g (7 oz) canned baked beans with pork sausages or 200 g (7 oz) baked beans and 1 egg fried in oil spray.

DINNER 125 g (4 oz) venison steak or 1 large mushroom, topped with 25 g (1 oz) cheese and grilled, served with red cabbage and 1 chopped apple stir-fried with 5–6 chopped new potatoes.

SNACKS/TREATS Choose any two from: 1 cheese string and 4 strawberries; 2 segments of chocolate orange; 2 cream crackers topped with 1 teaspoon lemon curd.

DAY SIX

BREAKFAST 2 lemon and raisin pancakes topped with strawberries and 1 teaspoon honey.

LUNCH 125 g (4 oz) chicken breast or 3 slices of vegetarian bacon, grilled and served in a bun spread with a little mashed avocado, served with 1 small corn on the cob.

DINNER 50 g (2 oz) pasta (dry weight), boiled and topped with 200 g (7 oz) any ready-made carbonara sauce, served with 2 small pieces of garlic bread and a large rocket salad.

SNACKS/TREATS Choose any two from: 1 small handful dried cranberries; 100 g (3½ oz) crème caramel; 1 sachet of soup in a cup with 1 rye cracker.

DAY SEVEN

BREAKFAST 2 eggs, scrambled and served with 50 g (2 oz) smoked salmon, with 200 ml (7 fl oz) any fruit juice on the side.

LUNCH 125 g (4 oz) roast turkey (or 1 large slice of marrow and 1 small roast sweet potato), served with 75 g (3 oz) stuffing, unlimited carrots and cabbage and a little gravy.

DINNER Salad made with 125 g (4 oz) shoulder ham or 1 boiled egg, lettuce, tomato, cucumber and 3 tablespoons low-fat coleslaw, served with 1 slice of granary bread.

SNACKS/TREATS Choose any two from: 125 g (4 oz) fromage frais; ½ scone with a scraping of low-fat spread; 5 pieces of dried papaya.

Keeping the weight off

IF YOU'RE NOW HAPPY WITH YOUR WEIGHT, THEN HOW CAN YOU MAKE SURE THAT YOU MAINTAIN IT? DEVELOPING SOME OF THE HABITS LISTED BELOW WILL INCREASE YOUR CHANCES OF KEEPING THAT WEIGHT OFF.

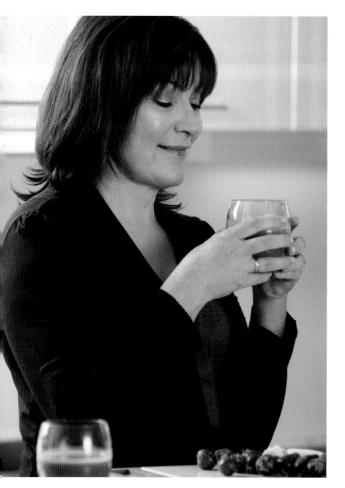

REASSESS YOUR EATING HABITS

If your body has changed, so too must your eating habits. The less you weigh, the fewer calories you burn throughout the day. In fact, on average, for every 500 g (1 lb) of fat you lose, you have to decrease your daily calorie intake by ten calories in order to keep your weight stable. Remember how you can calculate the number of calories you need in a day in order to maintain your weight (see page 23). Either use this method to determine your new healthy intake or stick to the eyeball method, which will naturally keep everything under control.

DON'T GIVE UP BREAKFAST

In every study ever carried out on successful slimmers, it's been found that breakfast eaters have an easier time maintaining their weight. Partly this is because breakfast revs up your metabolism so you burn maximum calories throughout the morning. Eating something healthy first thing, makes you less likely to reach for sugary snacks come 11 am.

USE THE 80:20 RULE

Nothing in moderation will make you fat – if you eat healthily 80 per cent of the time, you can eat what you want for the other 20 per cent without gaining weight. You can decide how you want to use this – for example, have two meals a week where you don't care what you eat or allow yourself one treat food every day. Whichever option you choose, be sure to enjoy it and don't feel guilty. Guilt tends to lead to binges and these do pile on the pounds.

WEIGH YOURSELF REGULARLY

According to the experts who compile the United States' National Weight Registry (which looks at the habits that successful slimmers use to keep the weight off) regular weigh-ins help you to spot weight gain early on, when it's easy to correct. The key to this is to set yourself a cut off point – agreeing to take action if you gain, say, 2 kg (4 lb). Remember, however, that weight can fluctuate daily (hormones, long flights, the weather and how much salt you ate the day before can all add fluid and, therefore, pounds). You only need to take action if you know the gain is part of an upward trend, or if it remains 3–4 days in a row following a big blowout, like a holiday.

EXERCISE

When US experts studied how people who've lost weight keep it off, they found that they do 60–90 minutes of exercise a day. This doesn't mean that they're permanently in the gym. Many of them do their workouts in 10–15 minute bursts of walking or running throughout the day. (See pages 90–117 for lots of suggestions on how to make exercise a part of your life.)

BEWARE OF OTHER PEOPLE'S REACTIONS

While you might be thrilled that you've lost weight, others might not be – friends can become jealous, partners can feel threatened – so watch out for sneaky saboteurs who might try to give you extra food.

Also look out for over-carers: people who ask whether you should really be eating one food or another after having worked so hard to lose

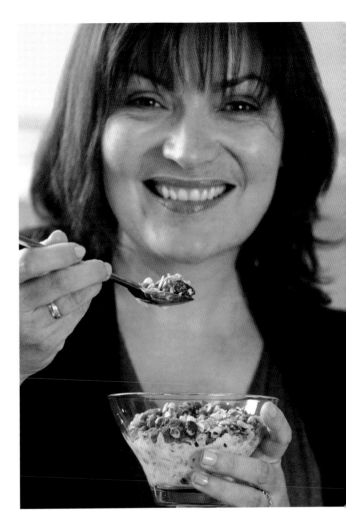

weight. They might think they're helping, but it may cause you to rebel and eat more of the food as you try to show that you know best.

STAY MOTIVATED

The day will come when people stop noticing that you have lost weight. This doesn't make it any less of an achievement, but it can be the time when your motivation starts to slip. If you need positive reinforcement, set yourself a new goal, such as learning to swim or running a 3-mile (5-km) race. This will keep your weight under control and give you the big mental 'cheers' you enjoy – and who knows, one day you might find yourself crossing the finishing line of a marathon or triathlon event.

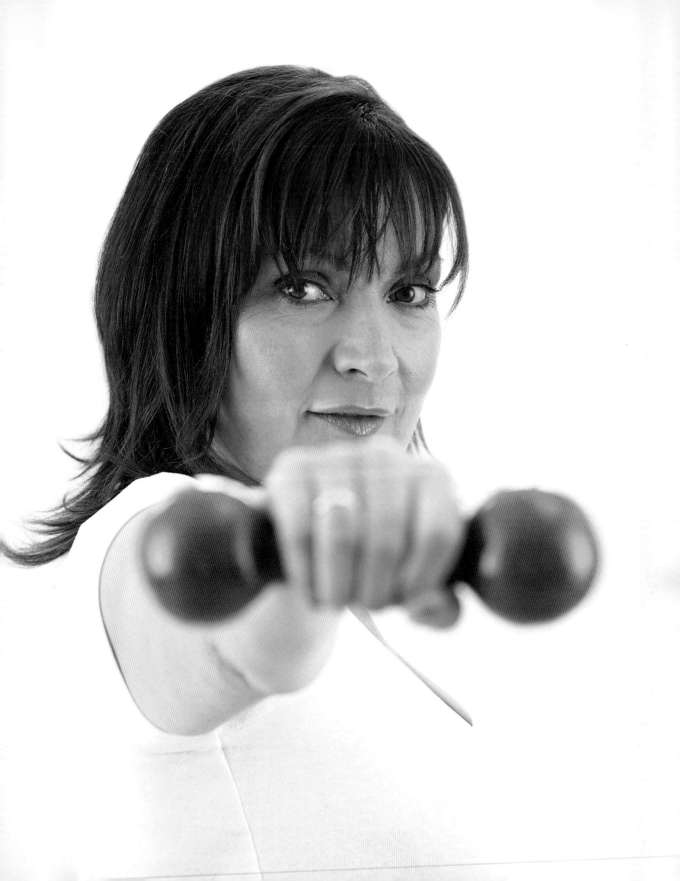

EXERCISE

Why exercise?

IT MIGHT SEEM ILLOGICAL BUT EXERCISE
ACTUALLY GIVES YOU ENERGY. I HAVE NEVER
FELT MORE ALIVE THAN WHEN I WAS
TRAINING FOR THE LONDON MARATHON AND,
ALTHOUGH I DON'T DO THAT MUCH EXERCISE
THESE DAYS, I DO FEEL BETTER WHEN I'VE
BEEN FOR A WALK OR DONE SOME PILATES.

GREAT FOR YOUR HEALTH

There are many excellent reasons for you to
exercise for the sake of your health. Regular
exercise offers all of the following benefits:

- Reduces risk of potentially serious health
  conditions, including heart disease, high blood
  pressure, osteoporosis and diabetes.
- Reduces overall risk of cancer.
- Increases levels of high-density lipoprotein
  (HDL), or 'good' cholesterol.
- Regulates hormone levels.
- Builds and maintains healthy muscles.
- Keeps joints, tendons and ligaments flexible,
  allowing you to move more easily (this is even
  more important as you get older).
- Helps you lose weight (teamed with a sensible
  diet) or, if you're already happy with your
  weight, helps you stay that way.

AND THERE'S MORE!

If the health benefits don't get you motivated,
there are plenty of other reasons to get out and
get active:

- Exercise makes you happy! Brain chemicals,
  such as serotonin and endorphins, which are
  released when you exercise, affect your mood.
  They relieve stress and depression, stimulate

feelings of euphoria and make you feel
invigorated.
- Recent studies suggest that exercise can reduce
  some of the effects of ageing. That alone is a
  great reason to take it up.
- Doing some regular exercise will build
  endurance and will give you extra energy –
  something that is really important to most
  busy women.
- Nothing else will tone and smooth those wobbly
  bits properly, making you look better and feel
  more self-confident.
- If you are active you're more likely to get a good
  night's sleep naturally.

HOW MUCH AND HOW OFTEN?

Some people are put off exercising because they
think it means playing sport or doing something
really vigorous, like running a marathon. But
you can gain enormous health benefits from
regular physical activity that doesn't involve
joining a gym or getting too red-faced and sweaty.
You just need to aim for at least 30 minutes of
moderate-intensity activity five days a week.
'Moderate intensity' means doing something that
increases your heart rate and makes you feel
warm, but that allows you to talk without panting.

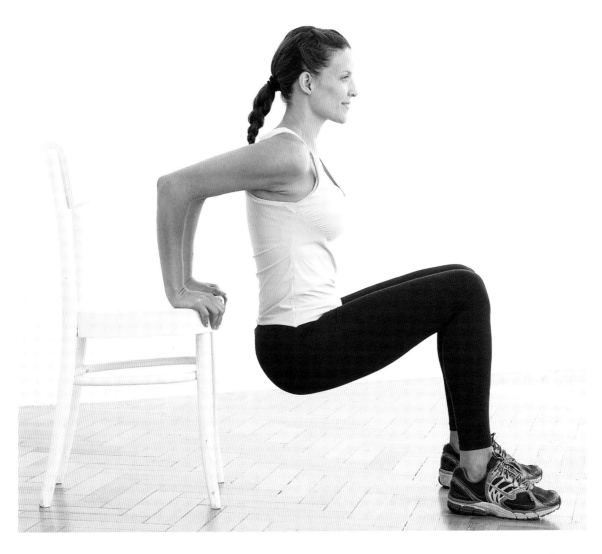

This could include, for example, walking briskly, mowing the lawn or doing some speedy vacuuming. If you're just starting to take regular exercise, you can build up to 30 minutes in two separate 15-minute sessions or three sessions each of 10 minutes.

One very easy way to get started is to follow the simple fitness programme that follows later on in this chapter (see pages 60–89).

THINK FIT

Adding 'hidden' exercise to your everyday routine is a clever way of keeping fit and staying active. For example, get into the habit of taking the stairs rather than the lift at work. Walk up the escalator. Park your car as far away as you can from the entrance to the supermarket to add a few more steps to your day. Another really good habit is to walk short distances instead of driving – you'll save petrol and use up calories at the same time.

Stop piling up things that need putting away at the bottom of the stairs – carry them up individually instead. It won't take long and there's nothing to beat climbing stairs for toning those thighs. Or you could challenge yourself to get the housework done in half the time and enjoy a workout while you're at it.

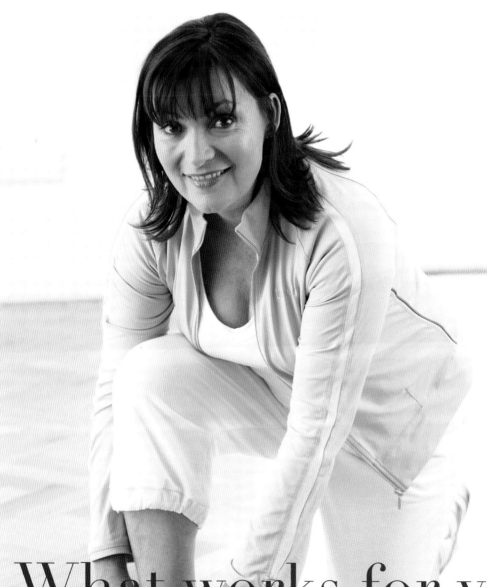

What works for you?

ALL EXERCISE IS GOOD FOR YOU, BUT
DIFFERENT TYPES – AEROBIC, FLEXIBILITY
AND STRENGTH EXERCISE – OFFER DIFFERENT
BENEFITS FOR YOUR BODY. I HAVE ALWAYS
BEEN LUCKY ENOUGH TO FIND EXERCISE
REGIMES THAT FIT IN WITH MY LIFESTYLE –
AND THAT I ACTUALLY ENJOY DOING.

AEROBIC EXERCISE

Aerobic or cardiovascular exercise raises your pulse and increases blood flow to your muscles. If done regularly and for at least 30 minutes at a time, this form of exercise will make your heart stronger and more effective at pumping blood. There are so many different options to try out – swimming, running, brisk walking, aerobics, circuit training or cycling, to name just a few!

FLEXIBILITY EXERCISE

This type of exercise includes yoga, t'ai chi and Pilates. It's all about stretching the muscles, making them more supple, and improving posture and breathing. A bonus is the sense of calm and wellbeing that flexibility training will bring you.

STRENGTH EXERCISE

This focuses on building up the size and strength of specific muscles. Strength exercise includes weightlifting, resistance training, such as aqua aerobics, and using variable-resistance machines at the gym.

WHAT WORKED FOR ME?

The most important thing about exercise is that you should enjoy it. Here's how I have made different types of exercise work for me:

Strutting my stuff When I was younger, I loved going to aerobics classes in Glasgow, although I was always the one at the very back who was two or three steps behind the rest of the class. The class was fun and the instructor had a terrific personality. She played some really good music, which had everyone giving their all.

Walking the dog I find going for a brisk 30-minute walk a terrific way to keep fit and it's a really good starting point for anyone who wants to tone up. I have a little Border terrier called Rocky who would walk all day if I let him. Come rain, snow or sunshine, he has to be walked and this means that I manage to get some activity every day.

Running for miles I ran the London Marathon in 2004 and did both the London and New York Marathons in 2005. If I can do it, anyone can, but you do have to put in the miles and stick to a training plan. Otherwise you risk serious injury and the disappointment of not completing the course. I've never been fitter, but it was a real commitment and, while I would not suggest that you start off by aiming for the ordeal of a 26-mile (42 km) run, I do think it is important to have some sort of goal when you are trying to get fit. This could be something simple like running for a mile without stopping or completing a circuit of the local running track or football pitch. Then, as you achieve each goal, you can set a new and more challenging one!

Body shaping I have now moved on to Pilates and I can thoroughly recommend this form of exercise. It looks deceptively simple but achieves really amazing results. Find out more about Pilates on pages 90–117.

ALL IN A GOOD CAUSE

Why not double the rewards of getting fit by helping a good cause at the same time? You can organize a sponsored run, walk or swim for charity or take part in an event like Race For Life, which is in aid of Cancer Research UK.

I've been doing the MoonWalk for the past seven years. This is a really incredible event, organized by the charity Walk the Walk, and raises millions of pounds for breast cancer research each year.

People taking part can sign up for the Full Moon (26 miles/42 km) or the Half Moon (13 miles/21 km). Everyone sets off at midnight and walks – no-one is allowed to run – through the night. All the women, and a handful of men, wear decorated bras – the crazier the better – and the atmosphere is extraordinary. It's a tough walk but all the camaraderie helps you to forget your tired legs.

What gets you through any fundraising event is the amount of money you can raise for your charity. That's worth all those blisters and aches and pains.

Let's get going!

THE HARDEST PART OF ANY EXERCISE
PROGRAMME IS TAKING THAT FIRST STEP.
IT'S ALL TOO EASY TO PUT THINGS OFF BY
MAKING A CUP OF TEA OR WATCHING TV.
TAKE BABY STEPS AT FIRST AND YOU WILL
BE AMAZED AT HOW QUICKLY YOUR BODY
CHANGES AND HOW GOOD YOU FEEL.

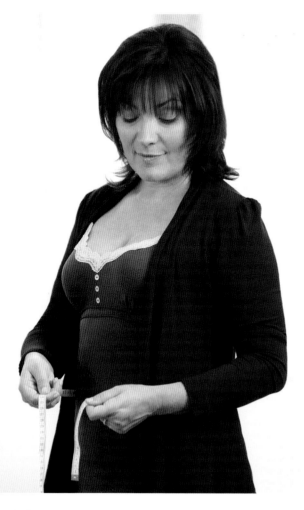

CHOOSING THE RIGHT EXERCISE FOR YOU

Anyone new to exercise should build up gradually
– whatever you do, don't be tempted to take on too
much, too soon. Also, you're much more likely to
stick to an exercise regime, be it rollerblading or
yoga, if you choose an activity that you enjoy and
something that you can realistically fit into your
lifestyle.

A class or a club is a great way to make new
friends so, if you fancy something sociable, look at
what's available in your area. Classes vary from
fencing to salsa, so you're bound to find something
to suit you.

On the other hand, you might need to be flexible
about when and where you exercise, in which case
something more independent, such as running,
swimming or a home-exercise DVD, would be ideal
for you.

Whatever option you choose, you need to plan
your exercise sessions in order to make sure that
you set aside the time you need every week, that
your sessions fit into your lifestyle, and that you
stay committed.

ASSESSING YOUR FITNESS

By recording some simple data before you begin
your programme, you will be able to assess just
how much you are progressing.

Body mass index (BMI) Your body mass index (see pages 34–35) is one measurement you can take to help you determine your success.

Waist–hip ratio (WHR) You can use your waist–hip ratio measurement to determine your body shape. Here's how it works: divide your waist measurement by your hip measurement. If the ratio is 0.8 or below, you are pear shaped; if it is greater than 0.8, you are apple shaped. Both men and women can be either shape.

The pattern of fat distribution throughout your body is an important predictor of health risks. An apple shape – where fat is stored around the midriff and gives the appearance of a heavy body with no waist definition – is considered to have a higher health risk from diabetes, heart disease, high blood pressure and stroke. A pear-shaped individual – where fat accumulates around the thighs, hips and bottom, is considered to be healthier.

Target heart rate (THR) Monitoring your heart rate during cardiovascular (aerobic) exercise can help you to exercise more efficiently. In order to get the best results from your workout, you should aim to work at 70–80 per cent of your maximum heart rate (MHR). Here's how to work it out: subtract your age from 220 – this is your MHR, in beats per minute. To find your THR, simply multiply your MHR by 0.7 (70 per cent) or 0.8 (80 per cent). So, for example, a 40-year-old woman will have an MHR of 180 beats per minute (220 minus 40). Seventy per cent of this gives a THR of 126 beats per minute; 80 per cent gives a THR of 144 beats per minute.

SMART EATING

A good exercise programme works best in conjunction with a healthy eating regime. This is because your weight is determined by the number of calories you eat in relation to the number of calories that you burn. Exercising will help you to burn more calories and you will achieve your goals that much more quickly if you eat a nutritionally balanced, healthy diet (see pages 8–51).

I HAVE FOUND THAT REGULAR EXERCISE IS GOOD FOR BOTH BODY AND SOUL

HOW MANY CALORIES ARE YOU BURNING?

We all burn up calories at different rates, depending on a number of factors. The calories listed here, therefore, are a guideline only. However, they will give you a pretty good idea of how many calories you can expend and whether you've done enough to justify an extra biscuit with your tea! This is based on a woman weighing 68 kg (10½ stone) and assumes a moderate effort.

Exercise	Average calories burned in an hour
Aerobics	440
Badminton	300
Canoeing and rowing	475
Circuit training	540
Cycling	540
Golf (pulling clubs)	290
Hockey	540
Horse riding	270
Jogging	475
Judo and karate	680
Kickboxing	680
Pilates	240
Skiing (downhill)	410
Softball	340
Squash	815
Swimming	470
Table tennis	270
T'ai chi	270
Tennis (doubles)	340
Tennis (singles)	540
Walking	225
Yoga	170

A simple fitness programme

YOU CAN ADAPT THIS SIMPLE FITNESS
PROGRAMME, DESIGNED BY EXERCISE AND
HEALTHCARE EXPERT SALLY LEWIS, TO SUIT
YOU. THE SOONER YOU START, THE MORE YOU
AND YOUR HEALTH WILL BENEFIT, SO WHAT
ARE YOU WAITING FOR?

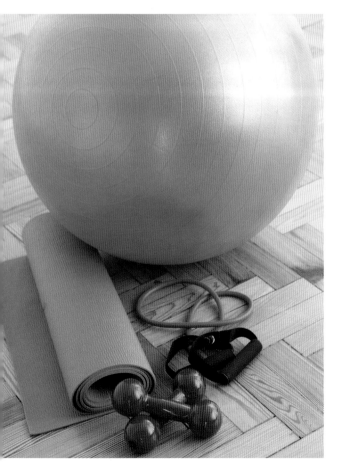

HOW THE PROGRAMME WORKS

The cardiovascular work helps you burn calories,
while the resistance work helps you to tone up and
burn calories. The flexibility section (warming up
and cooling down) makes sure you keep your
joints, ligaments and muscles supple.

Say you choose programme 1. You will spend 25
minutes working out each day (excluding warming
up and cooling down) for five to six days of the
week. For programme 3, with a 50-minute daily
workout, you'll find that three to four sessions a
week are sufficient for good results.

After six months, review the measurements
that you took at the start of the programme and
see what your results are. You may find that you
can continue with the programme you have
chosen, or that you need to change to another
programme in order to boost your results.

SET YOUR GOALS

Most people start a new fitness regime full of
enthusiasm, but after just a few weeks many may
find their motivation lacking. Generally, if you set
your targets too high to begin with, or exercise too
much initially, you soon lose interest. That's why
it's so important to set specific and realistic goals.

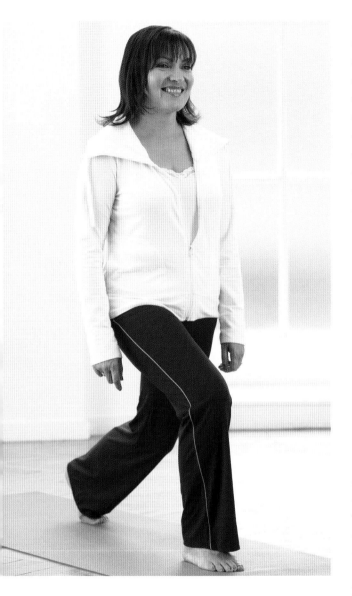

WHICH PROGRAMME?

There are several versions of the fitness programme to choose from – see which one suits you best. Remember: start easy and build up gradually. Warming up and cooling down before and after any exercise programme is essential to avoid injury, but bear in mind that warm-up and cool-down times are in addition to the overall programme time.

The four programmes:

Programme 1 / Five to six sessions per week/ 15 minutes of cardiovascular work, followed by 10 minutes of resistance work.

Programme 2 / Four to five sessions per week / 20 minutes of cardiovascular work, followed by 20 minutes of resistance work.

Programme 3 / Three to four sessions per week / 30 minutes of cardiovascular work, followed by 20 minutes of resistance work.

Programme 4 / Three sessions per week / 30–45 minutes of cardiovascular work, followed by 20–30 minutes of resistance work.

STAYING MOTIVATED

This is all about positive thinking and remembering why you started in the first place. When you'd rather stay in and watch TV you need to focus on exactly why you are going for that run or to the gym. Think of yourself wearing a swimsuit without having to wrap a sarong around yourself or imagine not having to resort to a kaftan to cover up your flabby arms.

It's a very good idea to enlist a family member or friend to join you at the class or on your daily run or walk. Neither of you will want to let the other down and having someone to talk to makes the time fly. I used to go training with my friend Joyce and we talked nonstop as we ran and walked; we solved all our problems, all our friends' problems and would probably have brought about world peace if we'd continued training to run marathons!

Don't just focus on your weight, think about how you want your body to look. A toned, more flexible body will make you look and feel fabulous.

One good practice is to set yourself a balance of short-term (weekly) goals as well as long-term ones (3–6 months). This way you get an extra boost every now and then as you tick them off your list. Make sure you think about these short-term goals carefully, however, as the more you know about what you want to achieve, the easier it will be to reach your targets.

Warming up

START YOUR WARM-UP BY DOING 5–10 MINUTES OF CARDIOVASCULAR EXERCISE, MAKING LARGE CONTROLLED ARM CIRCLES OR SIMPLY PUMPING YOUR ARMS AS YOU DO THEM. THEN DO THE FOLLOWING STATIC STRETCHES. IF YOU DO FEEL DISCOMFORT THEN EASE OFF THE STRETCH A LITTLE.

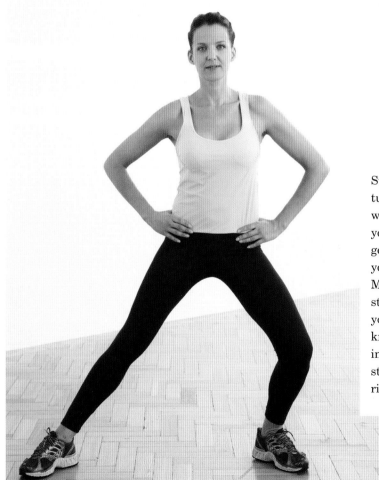

INNER THIGH AND GROIN STRETCH

For the best effects, keep your stomach pulled in towards your spine.

Stand upright with your feet turned slightly out and double hip-width apart. Place your hands on your hips and, breathing out, gently bend your left knee, taking your body weight over to the left. Make sure you keep your back straight and do not lean forward as you stretch. Do not allow your left knee to go over your toes. Breathe in and push back up to your starting position. Repeat on the right side.

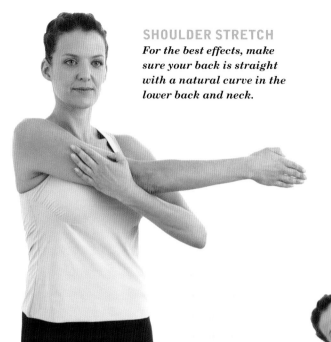

SHOULDER STRETCH

For the best effects, make sure your back is straight with a natural curve in the lower back and neck.

Place your right arm across the front of your body and, using your left hand, hold your right arm just above the elbow. Gently pull your right arm across and close to your body without twisting. Remember to keep your shoulders down and to breathe as you hold the stretch. You will feel the stretch in your shoulder and in your chest area. Repeat with your left arm.

SIDE STRETCH

For the best effects, make sure you keep your shoulders relaxed and down.

Stand with your arms resting down by your sides. Breathe out and slide your right hand down the side of your right leg, allowing your head to drop over to the right shoulder. Stretch your fingers downwards and make sure you pull in your stomach muscles to maximize the stretch. Breathe in, and return to your starting position. Repeat down the left-hand side.

Neck and shoulder exercises

THESE EXERCISES WILL HELP TO KEEP YOUR NECK MOBILE, WORK YOUR SHOULDERS AND STRNGTHEN YOUR UPPER BACK.

LATERAL RAISE

You can perform this exercise using either resistance bands or small hand weights. Keep your arms straight throughout the exercise – but don't lock your elbows – and keep your shoulders down.

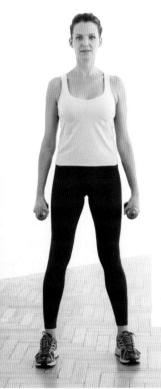

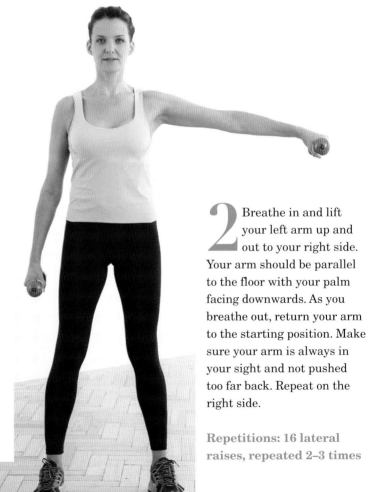

1 Stand with your feet hip-width apart, stomach pulled in and shoulders relaxed and down. You should have a natural curve in the lower back and neck areas. Hold a dumbbell in each hand, arms down by your sides.

2 Breathe in and lift your left arm up and out to your right side. Your arm should be parallel to the floor with your palm facing downwards. As you breathe out, return your arm to the starting position. Make sure your arm is always in your sight and not pushed too far back. Repeat on the right side.

Repetitions: 16 lateral raises, repeated 2–3 times

OVERHEAD PRESS WITH TWIST

Use small hand weights for this exercise, which will work your shoulders and your arms.

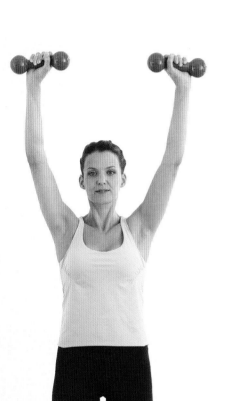

1 Sit or stand with a dumbbell in each hand and with your elbows bent so that your palms are directly in front of your shoulders.

2 Straighten your elbows and push the dumbbells upwards, above your head.

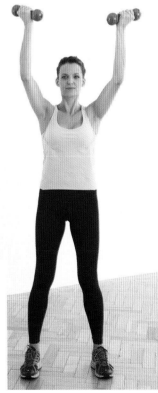

3 Twist your hands so that your palms now face outwards. Lower your arms, twisting your palms to face in again.

Repetitions: 16 overhead press with twist, repeated 2–3 times

Arm exercises

THESE EXERCISES WILL STRENGHTEN YOUR MUSCLES, TONE UP YOUR ARMS AND HELP TO BANISH 'BINGO WINGS'.

TRICEP DIP

The aim of this exercise is to tighten the muscle at the back of your arm, giving tone and shape to the arms. It is your arms that should be working here, so don't use your legs or back to push you up. You can do this exercise on a chair, bench, step or even on the edge of your bed.

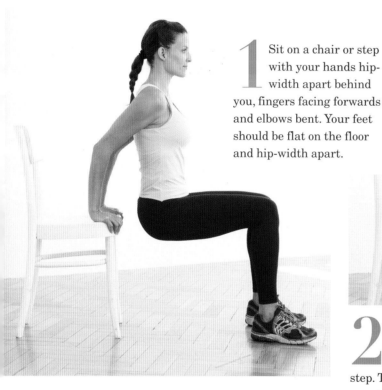

1 Sit on a chair or step with your hands hip-width apart behind you, fingers facing forwards and elbows bent. Your feet should be flat on the floor and hip-width apart.

2 Pull in your stomach and, keeping your back straight, lift your body weight up and off the chair or step. Then, bending your elbows, lower your bottom towards the floor. Make sure your elbows remain pointing backwards. Push yourself back up using your arms. Remember to keep your back straight. Lower back down and repeat.

Repetitions: 16 dips, repeated 2–3 times

TEACHER'S TIP

To increase the intensity of this exercise, extend both feet straight out in front of you.

BICEP CURL WITH RESISTANCE BAND

The aim of this exercise is to strengthen and shape the main bicep muscle at the front of the upper arm. Keep your shoulders back and down while you perform the exercise. As you increase your strength, you can increase the resistance of the band. If you prefer, you can use light hand weights instead of the resistance band.

1 Stand with your feet hip-width apart, stomach pulled in and shoulders down. Place the resistance band under the soles of your feet (if your band is not very long place only one foot on it), holding the band in your hands with your palms facing upwards and your arms down by your sides.

2 Flexing your elbows, pull the band up towards your shoulders, keeping your elbows close to your sides. Gently squeeze the shoulder blades together as you bring your arms upwards. Hold for a second or two, then lower the band back to the starting position.

Repetitions: 16 bicep curls, repeated 2–3 times

TEACHER'S TIP

You can perform this exercise one arm at a time. If you do this, repeat the exercise 16 times on one side before changing the band over to the other hand.

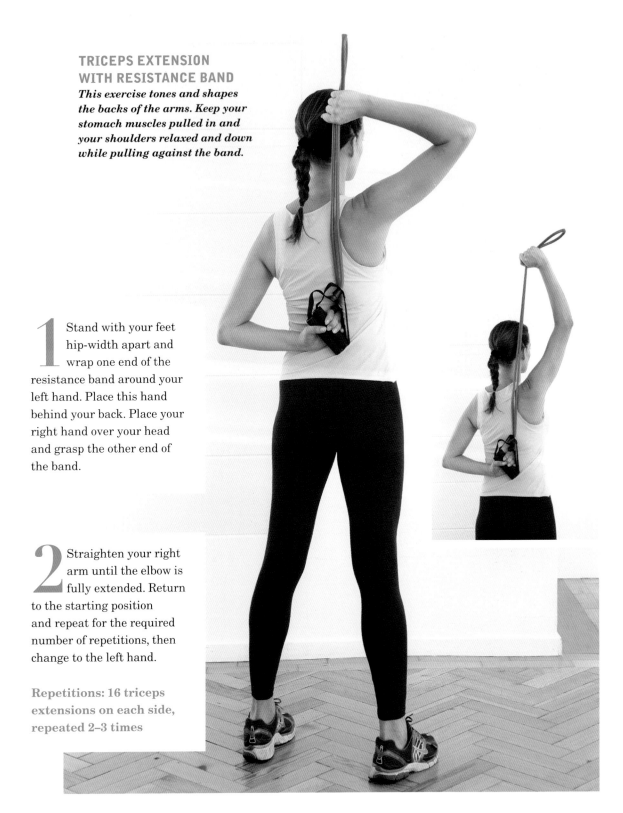

TRICEPS EXTENSION WITH RESISTANCE BAND

This exercise tones and shapes the backs of the arms. Keep your stomach muscles pulled in and your shoulders relaxed and down while pulling against the band.

1 Stand with your feet hip-width apart and wrap one end of the resistance band around your left hand. Place this hand behind your back. Place your right hand over your head and grasp the other end of the band.

2 Straighten your right arm until the elbow is fully extended. Return to the starting position and repeat for the required number of repetitions, then change to the left hand.

Repetitions: 16 triceps extensions on each side, repeated 2–3 times

PRESS-UP

Not only does this exercise strengthen your arms, but it also works the chest, back and abdominal muscles. Keep your stomach muscles tight during the whole exercise. Don't push up using your bottom or your back.

TEACHER'S TIP

If you want to make this exercise harder, extend your legs straight out behind you, hip-width apart. Keep your stomach tight, bend your elbows and lower your body and chest down towards the mat, then press back up.

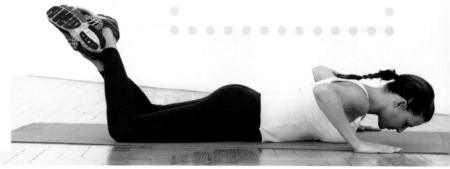

1 Lay on a mat, face down with your knees bent and your ankles crossed, your hands flat on the mat each side of your chest and slightly wider than shoulder-width apart.

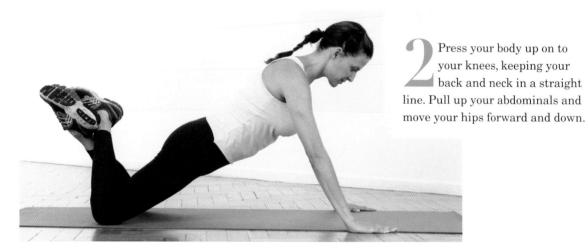

2 Press your body up on to your knees, keeping your back and neck in a straight line. Pull up your abdominals and move your hips forward and down.

3 Lower your chest towards the mat by bending your elbows, but make sure your chest does not touch the mat. Repeat for the specified number of repetitions, breathing in as you dip down and breathing out as you push back up.

Repetitions: 16 press-ups, repeated 2–3 times

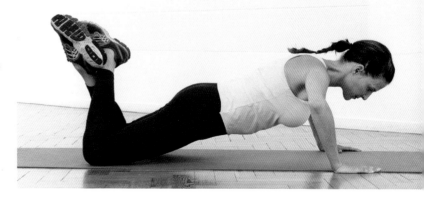

Back exercises

WITH THREE AREAS TO TARGET, INCLUDING
THE SIDE OF THE BACK, THE UPPER BACK
AND THE LOWER BACK, IT IS IMPORTANT TO
MAKE SURE YOU TRAIN EVERY AREA TO GET
THE BEST FROM YOUR WORKOUT.

DUMBBELL ROW

This exercise works the latissimus dorsi muscle on the back, stretching down from the armpit to the gluteal muscles. Working this muscle helps to define and shape the back. Keep your stomach muscles tight and draw your belly button back to the spine throughout the exercise.

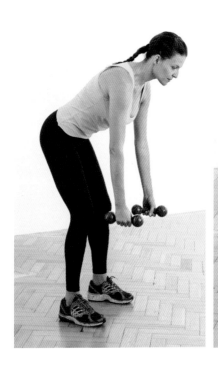

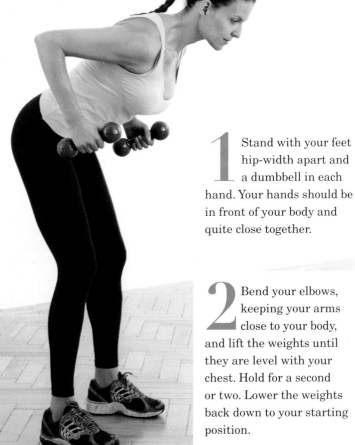

1 Stand with your feet hip-width apart and a dumbbell in each hand. Your hands should be in front of your body and quite close together.

2 Bend your elbows, keeping your arms close to your body, and lift the weights until they are level with your chest. Hold for a second or two. Lower the weights back down to your starting position.

Repetitions: 16 dumbbell rows, repeated 2–3 times

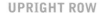

UPRIGHT ROW

This exercise helps to tone your upper back by working the trapezius and rhomboid muscles. Keep your stomach pulled in and your back straight throughout the exercise. Make sure you do not lift your shoulders as you lift your arms.

1 Stand with your feet hip-width apart, and with a dumbbell in each hand. Bend forward from your waist until your body is parallel to the floor (at a 45 degree angle), knees slightly bent. With your arms straight, but not locked at the elbow, hold the weights straight down towards the floor.

2 Bend your elbows and pull the weights up towards your hips, until your elbows are level with your body and parallel to the floor. Remember to keep your back flat and your shoulders relaxed. Return the weights back down towards the ground.

Repetitions: 16 upright rows, repeated 2–3 times

SEATED ROW WITH RESISTANCE BAND

This exercise is a good strengthening and toning exercise for the back, the shoulders and the abdominal muscles. It also helps to improve your posture. In order to be effective, you must keep your stomach muscles pulled in throughout the exercise and your shoulders must be over your hips throughout. Do not rush the exercise – focus on the muscles you are working.

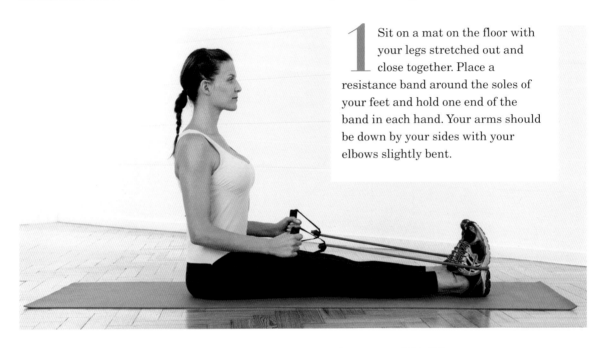

1 Sit on a mat on the floor with your legs stretched out and close together. Place a resistance band around the soles of your feet and hold one end of the band in each hand. Your arms should be down by your sides with your elbows slightly bent.

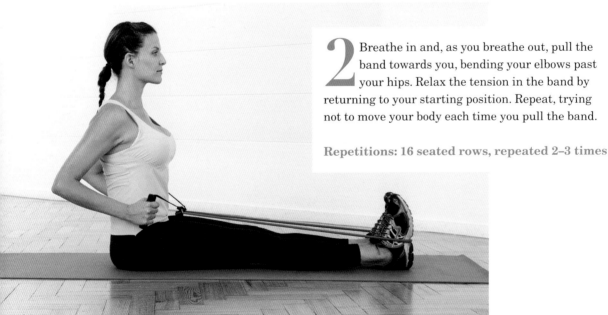

2 Breathe in and, as you breathe out, pull the band towards you, bending your elbows past your hips. Relax the tension in the band by returning to your starting position. Repeat, trying not to move your body each time you pull the band.

Repetitions: 16 seated rows, repeated 2–3 times

BACK EXTENSION

This exercise really works the lower back, helping to strengthen and stretch your back. Try to lengthen your back as you lift your chest up from the floor and press your shoulders down.

TEACHER'S TIP

If you want to increase the intensity of this exercise, lift your chest and both legs off the mat at the same time. Keep your legs straight and your pubic bone on the floor as you lift.

1 Lie face down on your mat, with your hands each side of your body or beside your head. Keep your legs together, flat on the floor.

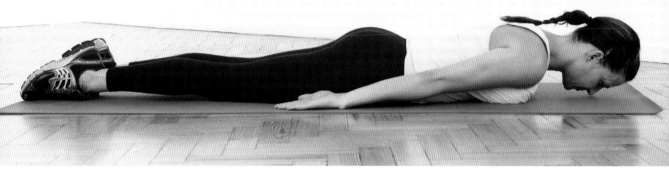

2 Pull in your stomach muscles and, as you breathe out, lift your chest off the mat. Try not to jerk the action. Breathe in as you return to your starting position.

Repetitions: 10 back extensions, repeated 2–3 times

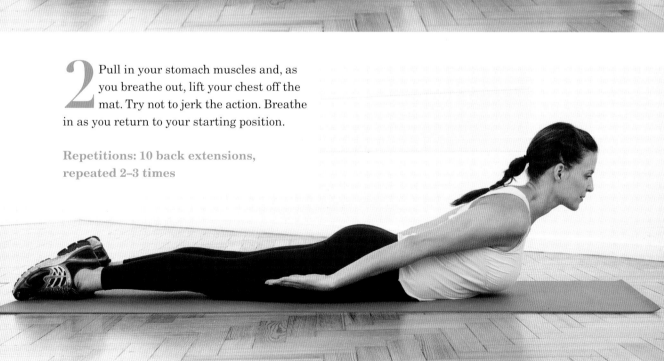

Chest exercises

THESE EXERCISES WILL STRENGTHEN AND TONE NOT ONLY YOUR CHEST BUT ALSO YOUR ABDOMINAL MUSCLES, BUTTOCKS AND LEGS.

DUMBBELL FLY
The exercise can also be performed without the ball, lying on a mat on the floor.

1 Lower your body on to the ball to get into the bridge position: the ball should be resting between your shoulders so that your lower back is clear of the ball; your feet should be hip-width apart, with your knees bent at 90 degrees and your hips lifted, so that they are in line with your knees and shoulders. Tighten your stomach muscles. Holding a dumbbell in each hand, bring them to your chest and hold them here.

2 Lift your arms straight up above your chest, palms facing, and bend your elbows so that the arms now form the shape of an arc.

3 Keeping the ball steady by controlling your stomach muscles, take the dumbbells out to each side, breathing in as you open your arms, and feeling the backs of your arms touch the sides of the Swiss ball. Breathe out as you push your arms and the dumbbells back up to your starting position. Remember to maintain the arc shape of your arms throughout the exercise.

Repetitions: 16 dumbbell flies, repeated 2–3 times

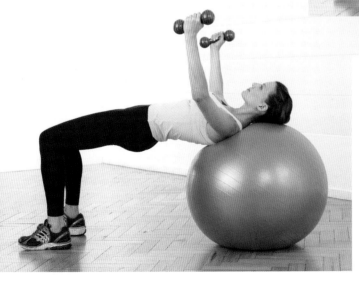

CHEST PRESS

This is a great exercise and can also be performed without the Swiss ball, lying on a mat on the floor. Keep your stomach muscles tight throughout the exercise and your shoulders relaxed.

1 Lower your body on to the ball to get into the bridge position: the ball should be resting between your shoulders so that your lower back is clear of the ball; your feet should be hip-width apart, with your knees bent at 90 degrees and your hips lifted, so that they are in line with your knees and shoulders. Tighten your stomach muscles. Holding a dumbbell in each hand, lift them up above the centre of your chest, and soften your elbows. Your palms should face outwards.

2 Breathe in as you lower the dumbbells, until you can feel the backs of your arms touch the Swiss ball.

3 Breathe out as you push the dumbbells back up. Remember to keep your bottom and hips lifted throughout the exercise, and your elbows soft and slightly bent.

Repetitions: 16 chest presses, repeated 2–3 times

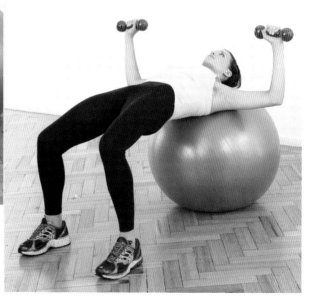

Waist exercises

THESE EXERCISE HELPS WHITTLE YOUR WAIST WHILE WORKING YOUR STOMACH MUSCLES TOO.

SIDE BRIDGE

Try to keep your shoulders relaxed, and pull your shoulder blades down as you lift your body up off the mat.

1 Lie on a mat in a straight line on your left side. Both legs should be together with your right foot lying on top of your left foot. Bend your left elbow beneath your left shoulder, placing your left forearm flat on the mat in front of you. Lay your right arm on your right leg.

TEACHER'S TIP

If you want to increase the intensity of this exercise, lift your top leg and arm up as you raise your body from the mat.

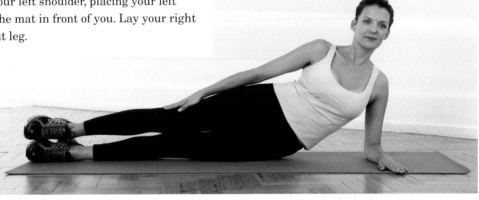

2 Lift your body up off the mat. Lower slowly back down to the starting position. Repeat on the right side.

Repetitions: 10 side bridges, repeated 2–3 times

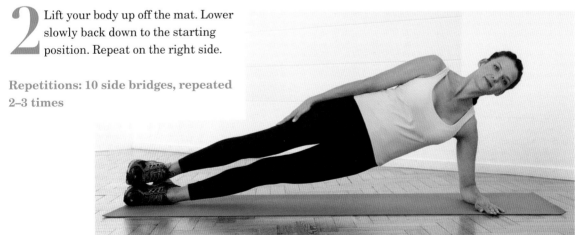

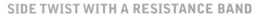

SIDE TWIST WITH A RESISTANCE BAND

This exercise targets your waist. Working with the band encourages a deeper stretch. Keep your posture throughout the exercise; your back should be straight, your stomach pulled in and your shoulders down. A straight back will always make you look longer and leaner.

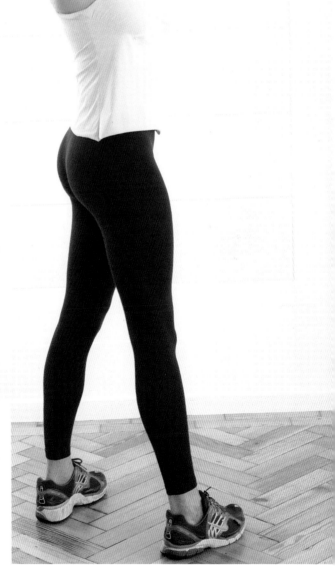

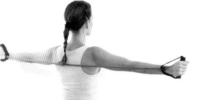

1 Stand with your feet hip-width apart and pass a resistance band around your back. Hold one end of the band in each hand and extend your arms straight out to the sides at shoulder height. Breathe in.

2 Turn to the right, keeping your arms straight and allow your head to follow the direction of the twist – to the right in this instance. As you twist, breathe out. Return to centre and repeat, this time turning to the left.

Repetitions: 16 side twists, repeated 2–3 times

Hip and thigh exercises

THESE EXERCISES HELP TO STRENGTHEN AND TONE YOUR THIGHS, GIVING YOU LEANER, LONGER, SEXIER LEGS.

PLIÉ

This classic dancer's exercise helps to tone and strengthen your legs. It works the hips, bottom, hamstrings and calves. Keep your knees over your toes, and your feet turned out at a 45-degree angle. Your back must be straight, with your stomach muscles pulled in.

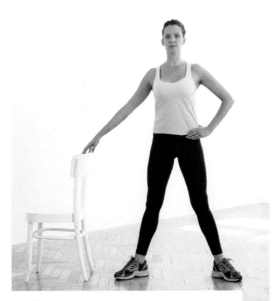

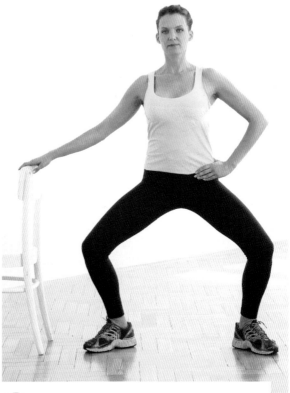

1 Hold on to the back of a chair with one hand. Stand with your feet slightly further than hip-width apart and your toes turned out. Breathe out and pull in your stomach, keeping your back straight and your shoulders pressed down and back.

2 Bend both knees, keeping your knees over your toes. Your thighs should be parallel to the ground. As you push down make sure your knees do not roll inwards and that your feet stay flat on the floor. Push back up to the starting position, and repeat.

Repetitions: 16 pliés, repeated 2–3 times

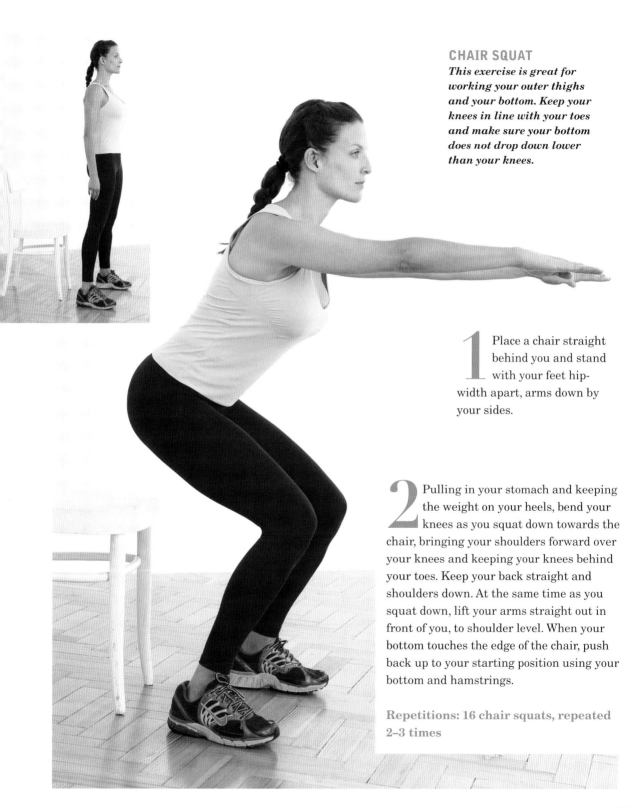

CHAIR SQUAT

This exercise is great for working your outer thighs and your bottom. Keep your knees in line with your toes and make sure your bottom does not drop down lower than your knees.

1 Place a chair straight behind you and stand with your feet hip-width apart, arms down by your sides.

2 Pulling in your stomach and keeping the weight on your heels, bend your knees as you squat down towards the chair, bringing your shoulders forward over your knees and keeping your knees behind your toes. Keep your back straight and shoulders down. At the same time as you squat down, lift your arms straight out in front of you, to shoulder level. When your bottom touches the edge of the chair, push back up to your starting position using your bottom and hamstrings.

Repetitions: 16 chair squats, repeated 2–3 times

INNER-THIGH LIFT

Working on the adductors – your inner thigh muscles – this exercise helps to strengthen and tone your thighs. Make sure your body is in a straight line as you lift your leg, and that your hips are aligned throughout the exercise.

1 Lie on your left side on a mat, left arm bent. Rest your head on your left hand. Your legs should be in a straight line from your body and your right hand placed on the floor in front of your right hip. Bend your right (top) knee and cross it over your left leg to place it flat on the mat (or, if you can, place your right foot flat on the mat).

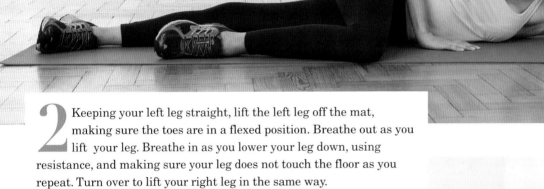

2 Keeping your left leg straight, lift the left leg off the mat, making sure the toes are in a flexed position. Breathe out as you lift your leg. Breathe in as you lower your leg down, using resistance, and making sure your leg does not touch the floor as you repeat. Turn over to lift your right leg in the same way.

Repetitions: 16 inner-thigh lifts, repeated 2–3 times

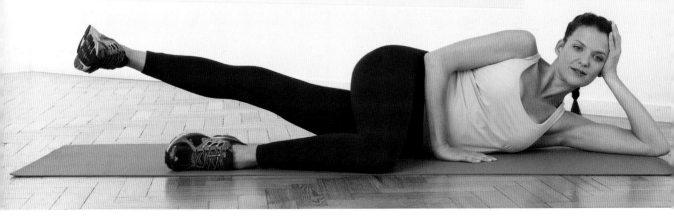

LYING SIDE LEG LIFT

This exercise strengthens your outer thigh muscles, the hips and buttocks, and your hip flexor muscles. Make sure you are lying in a straight line for this exercise; your shoulders and hips should be in line with your shoulders.

1 Lie on your left side in a straight line, with your left elbow bent and your left hand supporting your head. Place your right hand in front of you flat on the mat near to the body for support.

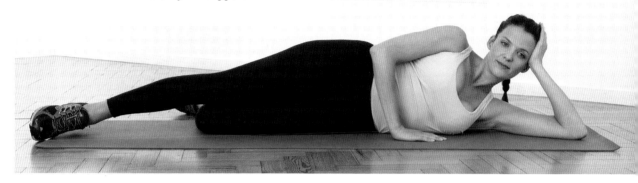

2 Bend your left knee underneath you and lift your right leg upwards, as high as you can, keeping your foot flexed. Breathe out as you lift and breathe in as you lower.

Repetitions: 16 lying side leg lifts, repeated 2–3 times

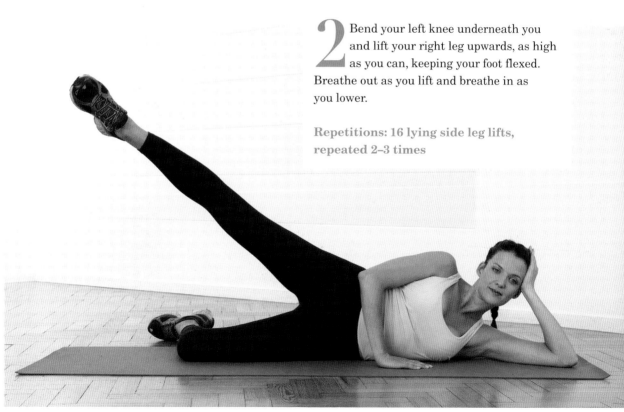

Bottom exercises

IF YOU WANT A PERT BUM THEN THESE
EXERCISES ARE FOR GREAT FOR TONING
AND LIFTING YOUR BOTTOM.

LUNGE

This is such a great exercise for toning your bottom. Keep your bent knee directly over your front foot, and your back knee straight throughout. Do not allow your body to move forward. You may find, at first, that you do not lower very far, but this will improve as you get stronger and fitter.

1 Stand with your feet approximately 90 cm (3 ft) apart and your hands on your hips. Take a large step forward with your left leg, making sure your right heel remains flat on the floor.

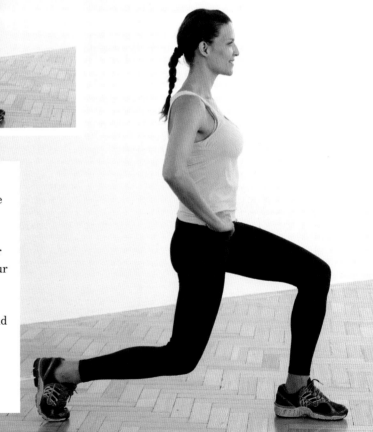

2 Bend your right knee and lower it straight down towards the floor, while lifting your right heel off the floor. Your left knee should be pointing straight ahead, with your left knee directly over your left foot. Keep your shoulders in line with your hips, so that you don't tip forward, and your stomach muscles pulled in. Push back up to your starting position, using your bottom and thigh, and repeat on your other leg.

Repetitions: 16 lunges on each leg, repeated 2–3 times

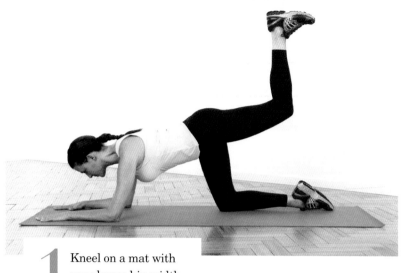

DONKEY KICK

This exercise certainly helps to tone and lift your bottom. Keep your pelvic floor and your stomach muscles pulled up throughout the exercise. You do not have to lift your leg high to activate your bottom muscles.

1 Kneel on a mat with your knees hip-width apart, and lower your chest towards the mat, resting on your forearms. Breathe out and pull your stomach muscles in towards your spine. Breathe in and lift your left leg up behind you towards the ceiling.

2 Flex your foot so the sole of your foot is facing upwards, towards the ceiling. Your left knee should be bent at 90 degrees, with your left hip and left knee in a straight line. Push your left leg upwards, squeezing your bottom.

TEACHER'S TIP

To increase the intensity of this exercise, use an ankle weight to perform the lift.

3 Bring your left leg back down towards the ground, keeping your knee bent, but do not let it touch the floor before repeating the exercise.

Repetitions: 16 donkey kicks on each knee, repeated 2–3 times

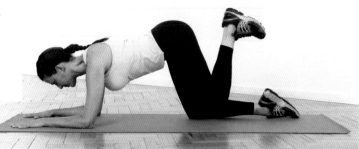

Leg exercises

THESE SIMPLE EXERCISES ARE DESIGNED TO HELP YOU BUILD STRENGTH AND GIVE SHAPE TO YOUR LEGS.

CALF RAISE

This exercise is a 'must' if you want to tone and shape the lower part of your legs. Keep your knees pulled up, but not locked, during the exercise. Keep your stomach muscles pulled up and your shoulders down.

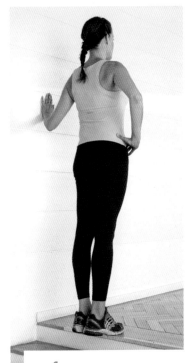

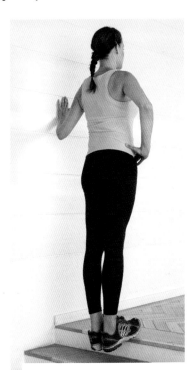

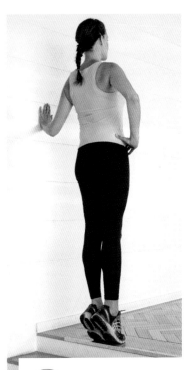

1 Stand with the balls of your feet on a step, book or even on the floor. Your feet should be slightly apart and your toes facing forwards. Place your hands on your hips, or hold on to the back of a chair, window ledge or a wall to help keep your balance.

2 Push your heels down as far as is comfortable (you will feel your calves stretch).

3 Keeping your knees straight, push up onto the balls of your feet, squeezing through your calves and your buttocks. Hold for a second or two then lower your heels back down.

Repetitions: 16 calf raises, repeated 2–3 times

LEG LIFT WITH A SWISS BALL

These exercises certainly give shape and strength to your legs. Keep your stomach muscles pulled in throughout the exercise, and your shoulders back and down. There should be no tension in your neck.

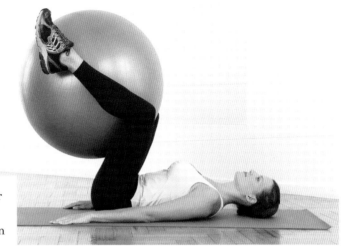

1 Lie on your back on a mat with your knees bent, and your arms by your sides. Pick up the Swiss ball between your ankles and lower legs by squeezing your legs together as you lift your knees just over your hips, towards your chest.

2 Sit up far enough to rest on your elbows.

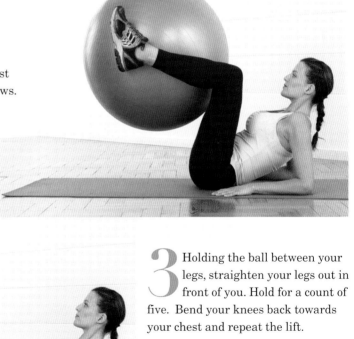

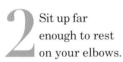

3 Holding the ball between your legs, straighten your legs out in front of you. Hold for a count of five. Bend your knees back towards your chest and repeat the lift.

Repetitions: 16 leg lifts, repeated 2–3 times

HAMSTRING ROLL

This exercise uses the Swiss ball to tone the legs, especially the hamstrings and the calves, at the same time working your stomach muscles and the lower back. Keep your stomach muscles pulled in and try not to drop your hips as you lift your bottom up.

1 Lie on your back with your legs straight and your heels resting on the Swiss ball. Your arms should be down by your side.

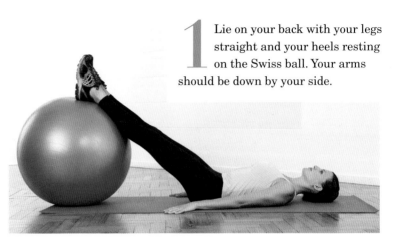

2 Slowly lift your bottom and your back up off the mat, keeping your body in a straight line from your shoulders to your feet.

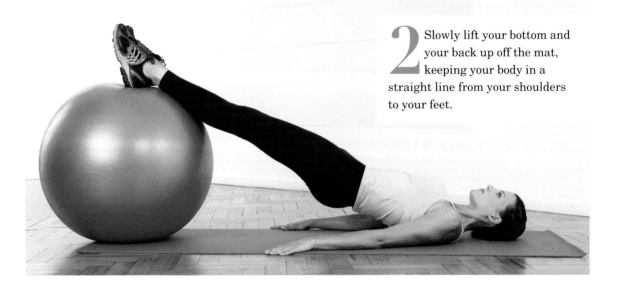

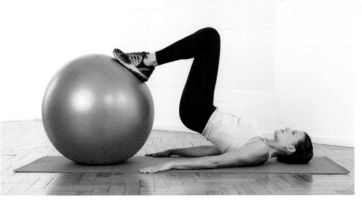

3 Squeezing the backs of your legs, roll the ball towards your bottom, breathing out and making sure you keep your hips lifted. Repeat, breathing out as you roll the ball towards you and breathing in as you roll the ball away.

Repetitions: 16 hamstring rolls, repeated 2–3 times

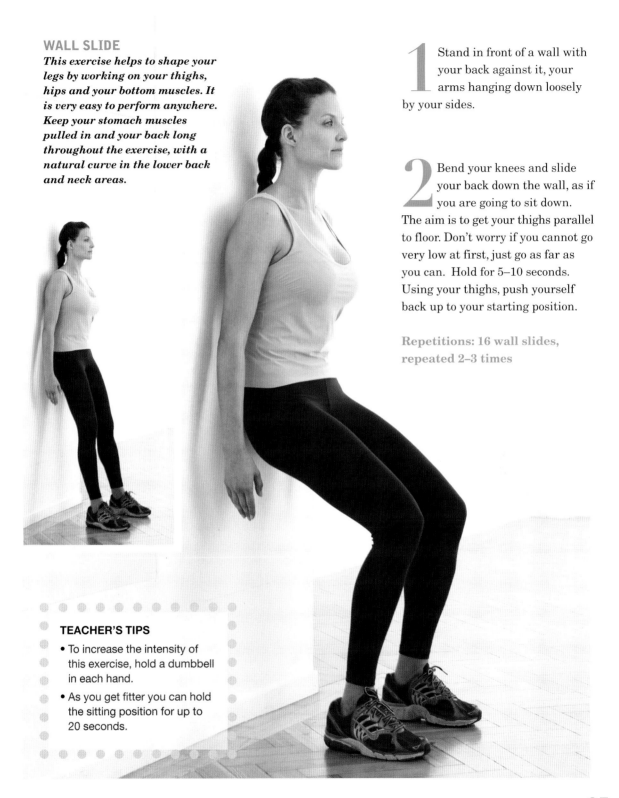

WALL SLIDE

This exercise helps to shape your legs by working on your thighs, hips and your bottom muscles. It is very easy to perform anywhere. Keep your stomach muscles pulled in and your back long throughout the exercise, with a natural curve in the lower back and neck areas.

1 Stand in front of a wall with your back against it, your arms hanging down loosely by your sides.

2 Bend your knees and slide your back down the wall, as if you are going to sit down. The aim is to get your thighs parallel to floor. Don't worry if you cannot go very low at first, just go as far as you can. Hold for 5–10 seconds. Using your thighs, push yourself back up to your starting position.

Repetitions: 16 wall slides, repeated 2–3 times

TEACHER'S TIPS

- To increase the intensity of this exercise, hold a dumbbell in each hand.
- As you get fitter you can hold the sitting position for up to 20 seconds.

Cooling down

DON'T SKIP THIS PART OF THE PROGRAMME, OR YOUR MUSCLES MAY FEEL SORE AND STIFF A DAY OR SO AFTER YOUR EXERCISE.

before you start your stretches spend a few minutes gently walking, to return your heart rate and breathing to normal. You can also use some of the warm-up stretches for cooling down (see pages 62–63). Hold each stretch for at least 10–30 seconds.

HAMSTRING STRETCH

For the best effects, make sure you pull in your stomach and lift forward from your hips as you perform this stretch.

CALF STRETCH

For the best effects, use a wall to help maximize this stretch.

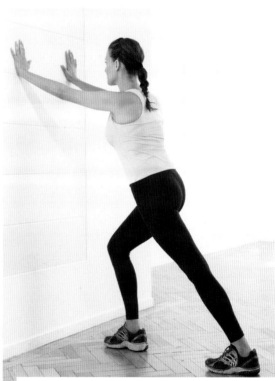

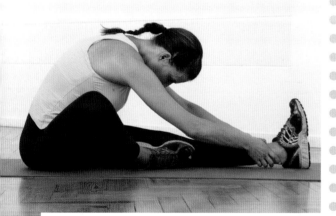

Sit on a mat with your left leg straight out in front of you, and your right leg bent. Place the sole of your right foot on the inside of your left thigh. Keeping your left foot flexed, lean forward from your hips, and slide your hands down your left leg towards your ankle. Breathe out as you stretch forward and feel the stretch in the back of your left thigh. Return to your starting position and repeat on your right leg.

Stand with your feet hip-width apart, back straight, stomach pulled in and shoulders down. Step backwards with your left foot, keeping the foot facing forwards. Bend your right knee, keeping it just behind your toes. Place your hands on the wall in front of you and push against it, keeping your heels on the floor. Feel the stretch in the calf of your right leg. Repeat with the right leg.

QUAD STRETCH

For the best effects, make sure you keep your knees in line.

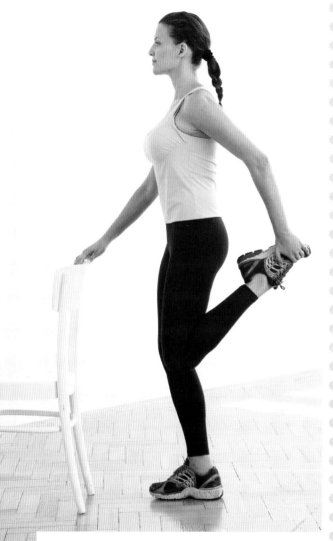

CAT STRETCH

For the best effects, slowly press your back down, vertebrae by vertebrae.

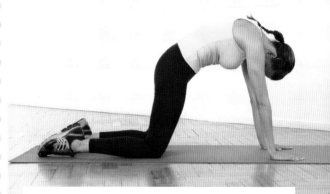

1 Kneel on all fours on a mat, with your legs hip-width apart, your feet pointing backwards and your hands under your shoulders and shoulder-width apart. Your fingers should face forwards. Breathe in and curl up through your back, tucking your head under and stretching your neck. Hold the stretch for a few seconds.

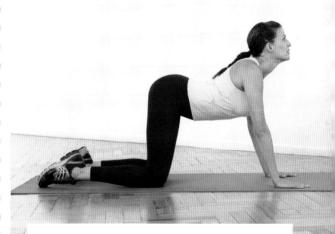

Stand in front of a wall or a chair, holding on with your right hand. Bend your left knee up behind you and grasp your foot with your left hand. At the same time make sure you keep a slight bend in your right knee. Pull your left heel towards your bottom, keeping your knees in line and pushing your hips forward. Feel the stretch in the front of your right thigh. Repeat on your right leg.

2 Release your breath, at the same time pushing down through your back so that it becomes concave. Continue the stretch through to your neck, so your head is up and you are looking towards the ceiling, lifting your chin.

Why I love Pilates

PILATES IS A WONDERFUL WAY TO BECOME FIT, SUPPLE AND TONED AT ANY AGE, AND IT CAN BE A GREAT FORM OF EXERCISE TO TAKE UP, EVEN IF YOU HAVE NEVER EXERCISED MUCH BEFORE. IF YOU DO IT PROPERLY YOU'LL REAP ENORMOUS BENEFITS.

WHAT IS IT?

Pilates exercises are based on the work of Joseph Pilates. Born in Germany, Pilates first developed his exercise method, which he called 'Contrology', in the early 1900s. Incorporating elements from martial arts, body-building and yoga, his exercises combined both Eastern and Western philosophies to create a holistic work-out. But it was out of the New York studio, in the late 1920s, that the Pilates Method we know of today was really defined. Athletes and ballet dancers flocked to his studio, and gradually the word spread. Pilates is now practised by millions of people around the world.

The Pilates Method is an exercise for both your mind and your body, which will improve your strength, flexibility and overall mobility to create a more balanced body. It is an exercise programme that builds core stability, along with strength and power of your trunk and limbs. Unlike some kinds of exercise, it won't bulk up your muscles to give a chunky look, but will elongate them as it strengthens them, to develop a more streamlined shape. Pilates improves your spinal flexibility, and your spinal

> PILATES IS MY FAVOURITE FORM OF EXERCISE AND HAS HELPED ME TO RELIEVE STRESS AND TO STAY AGILE

and joint mobility too. As a result, you will find your posture will change, your body will start to move more efficiently, and you'll improve your overall appearance.

MIND–BODY CONNECTION

The method is a holistic one, and requires you to focus your mind on individual muscles in order to strengthen and lengthen them. As you move, this concentration and precision creates a mind–body connection, the mental focus encouraging the muscles to work to the maximum, so that you get faster and better results.

Because Pilates helps you to get in tune with both your mind and your body, it is also relaxing: instead of feeling wiped out, as you do after a run or an aerobics class, you feel rested and revitalized after a Pilates session.

WHAT I LIKE ABOUT IT

Pilates is a wonderfully effective way to tone up and feel healthier, stronger and fitter. It's also a brilliant stress buster. If you look at anyone doing Pilates you might think it is an easy option, but if you do the exercises properly your body will

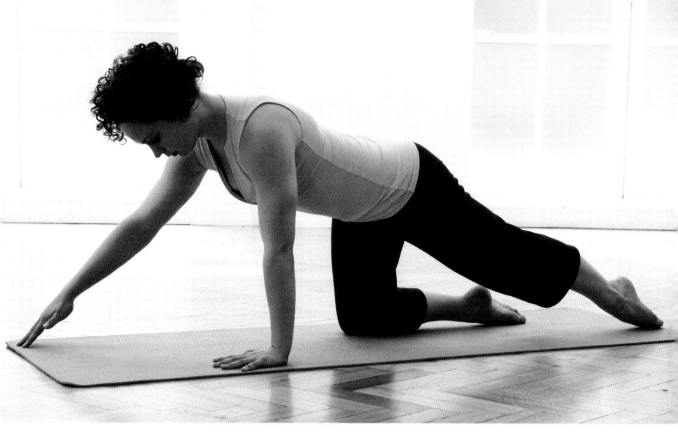

undergo a thorough, but very safe, work-out. You need to put in the effort to get the technique right, to ensure that you get the maximum benefits from the exercises.

Pilates does not involve stress or strain on your body – you won't be grunting, red-faced and panting at the end of a session – but you will still feel as though you have worked hard. You will actually notice a real difference in a relatively short space of time. Your posture will improve and your muscles will begin to firm and tone up.

WHO'S IT FOR?

Pilates is ideal for almost everyone, regardless of age, level of fitness and physical ability. Osteopaths, physiotherapists and GPs recommend Pilates as one of the safest methods of exercise around today, and under supervision by a qualified teacher, it can be highly beneficial for people with conditions like back pain and arthritis. Pilates pregnancy classes also offer a safe, gentle exercise option for pregnant women.

WHAT PILATES CAN DO FOR YOU

- Give you longer, leaner muscles.
- Give you a toned body with a flatter stomach, slimmer thighs and a smaller waistline.
- Strengthen your body and build core stability.
- Improve your flexibility.
- Improve the mobility of your spine and allow you to move more freely.
- Build better balance and coordination.
- Relieve a variety of minor aches and pains.
- Improve your posture.
- Improve your game and prevent injury if you're a sports enthusiast.
- Maintain and improve bone density to help you fight osteoporosis.
- Boost your immune system and improve your circulation.
- Enhance your sense of wellbeing.
- Reduce stress and tension.

A beginners' Pilates programme

THE FOLLOWING PAGES DESCRIBE TEN OF MY FAVOURITE BEGINNER'S PILATES EXERCISES, PUT TOGETHER BY PILATES FOUNDATION TEACHER, JENNIFER DUFTON.

this programme teaches you how to work from your centre, to build core stability and strength, and I cannot recommend a better way to start. All you need is a padded, nonslip exercise mat to protect your spine, and a folded hand towel or small flat pillow to support your

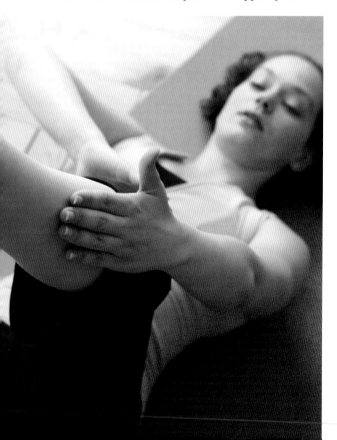

head, as shown in some of the exercises. Practise the exercises in the order shown, skipping any that feel too challenging for the time being. You can always return to them, once your core stability, strength and mobility have improved.

TAKE IT SLOWLY

Please, please don't be tempted to rush straight into these exercises. It is really important to read through the Pilates Basics section on pages 94–97 so that you lay down proper foundations first. Pilates is all about the quality of your movement, and you need to incorporate these fundamental techniques into all of the exercises to really reap the benefits.

Aim to practise the exercises three times per week. They will give you a good introduction to Pilates and each session will take approximately 15 minutes to perform. Also, as you work through them, monitor each movement – it is the attention to detail in Pilates that will change your body and your quality of life.

SAFETY FIRST

As with any exercise regime, the following exercises are only suitable if you are in good health, with no injuries or medical conditions that would prevent you from undertaking a Pilates programme. Take my advice: it is essential to consult your GP before starting if you have any injuries or health concerns, and especially if you are pregnant, have given birth in the last six weeks, or have a medical condition, such as high blood pressure, arthritis, osteoporosis or asthma. All matters regarding your health require medical supervision.

Also, while exercising, be especially aware of your body and how you are feeling. It is vital that you distinguish between effort and pain. An exercise may require effort to perform, but you should never feel you are straining in any way. If something hurts, or just doesn't feel right, stop and seek further advice.

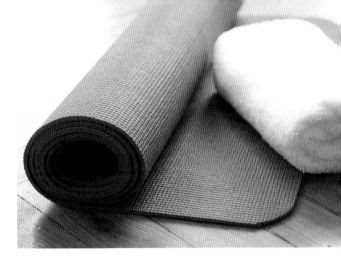

FINDING A TEACHER

You can use the exercises in this book to get started and to see what Pilates is all about. If you like it, and like the rewards of your efforts, you will need to progress to classes with a qualified teacher, who will help you to improve your technique and pinpoint any imbalances you may have. Taking Pilates classes with a teacher will also ensure that your exercise programme remains challenging and fun.

CORE STABILITY AND CORE STRENGTH

One of the principles upon which Pilates is founded is 'centring' – the idea being that all movement starts from your centre.

You may already know that there is a large cylinder of muscles in the centre of your body, which starts with the pelvic floor muscles, and includes muscles of the hips, stomach and back. Joseph Pilates called these muscles the 'powerhouse'. Nowadays we refer to this cylinder as our 'core' and, in line with the latest scientific research, it has expanded to include muscles further up the trunk. Your 'core' muscles link to your limbs via your pelvis and shoulders, and they also link the head and neck.

If they are weak, inflexible or stuck in habitual patterns, your core muscles can stop working

effectively, or cause restrictions, sometimes with painful results. Plus, if they aren't working properly, other muscles often try to take over. These tend to be the more superficial muscles that move your body, which can then overdevelop, or become overemphasized instead, causing further problems.

Pilates is all about addressing such imbalances by finding your core. In doing so you will create the stable, strong, yet pliable body you need for it to function at its very best. Core stability and core strength are vital. You need stability for a supportive core, which in turn will lead to a more stable pelvis and shoulders. You also need to strengthen your core, for your body to function most efficiently.

GREAT FOR YOUR HEALTH

This holistic exercise method offers many other benefits. Pilates is about breathing well, and improving mobility in your joints and spine. It's about restoring good alignment and posture. It's about building power and strength in your trunk and limbs. It's only when your body is functioning as an integrated whole, that you will truly look and feel great.

These exercises will set you on the path to achieving that balanced body. But you can't just do one session and forget about Pilates for the rest of the week if you want the best results. Pilates is about teaching your body to move well, so that you carry this knowledge with you in daily life.

Pilates basics

THERE ARE A COUPLE OF BASIC TECHNIQUES THAT YOU NEED IN ORDER TO GAIN THE MAXIMUM BENEFITS FROM THIS PROGRAMME. READ OVER THE INSTRUCTIONS ON PAGES 94–97 AND PRACTISE THE EXERCISES A FEW TIMES BEFORE YOU BEGIN.

RELAXATION POSITION

The Relaxation Position, with a neutral pelvis and neutral spine, is the start and finish position for many of the Pilates exercises that you perform lying down. It is important to get this position right, as you often need to maintain your neutral pelvis and neutral spine positions while performing the exercises. Here's how to find 'neutral pelvis'. Please note, in the photographs below the arms are positioned a little wider than usual so that you can see the position of the spine. When you are lying in the Relaxation Position, place your arms closer to your sides, with your hands in line with your shoulders.

1 Lie on your back on the mat with your knees bent, feet hip-width apart and in parallel. Place a small folded towel under your head. Nod your head forward slightly to lengthen the back of your neck. Your head should neither tip forward nor backwards. Place your arms by your sides, with your shoulders relaxed and your palms down. Tilt your pelvis up, by rocking your pubic bone up towards your navel. Your pelvis should tuck under, your waist should flatten and the gap between your lower back and the mat should be lost as your tailbone lifts off the mat.

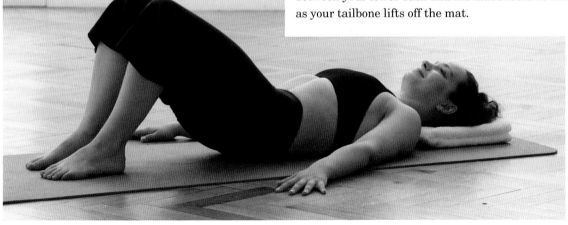

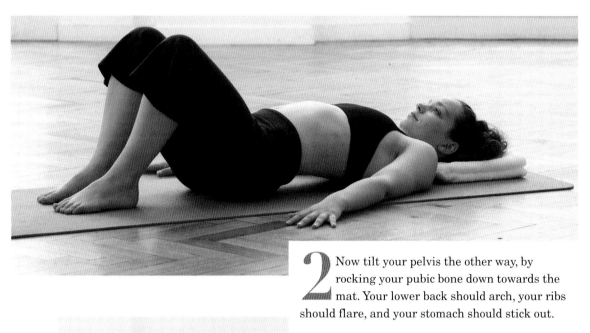

2 Now tilt your pelvis the other way, by rocking your pubic bone down towards the mat. Your lower back should arch, your ribs should flare, and your stomach should stick out.

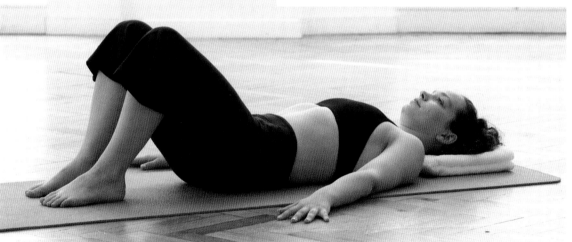

3 Neutral pelvis lies midway between these two positions. When you are 'in neutral', your two hip bones (at the front of your pelvis) lie in exactly the same plane as your pubic bone, so that they are all level. You should also be able to feel your sacrum resting squarely on the mat. Everyone's position will be slightly different, but with most people there is just enough room to slip a hand in the slight gap under their waist, when they are in neutral pelvis. Now bring your awareness to your spine in order to find neutral spine. If you were to change the angle of your pelvis, you would change the curves of your spine. Instead, remain in neutral pelvis as you try to lengthen your spine while maintaining the natural S-shape of your spine's curve. Allow the weight of your head, the back of your ribcage and the back of your pelvis to sink into the mat, and imagine your tailbone is lengthening away from you. You will now have a neutral spine.

LATERAL BREATHING

All the Pilates exercises in this programme use a particular kind of Pilates breathing, called lateral breathing, which encourages good function of the stabilizing muscles within your core. Breathing well oxygenates the blood and nourishes your body's cells, as well as expelling toxins and improving your circulation and skin tone. This style of breathing is the basic method for Pilates breathing. It has been kept deliberately simple because you are practising at home and therefore don't have the benefit of supervised instruction. Of course, there are many different styles of breathing, and a good Pilates teacher may teach you to breathe slightly differently if this would be of greater benefit to you.

Lorraine's tip

I found breathing this way felt a little different to start with, but it came with practice. When breathing out, I found it helpful to visualize my stomach muscles as a wide sheet of muscle covering my whole abdomen, starting just beneath my ribcage and extending all the way down to my pubic bone. Doing this ensures that you draw in the whole sheet, as it were, instead of focusing on just one small portion of it.

TEACHER'S TIP

• When performing the exercises in this programme, every time you read 'breathe out and stabilize', you should return to the 'breathe out' stage described opposite.

• Each time you breathe in, try not to take in huge amounts of air or you may begin to feel dizzy. All you need is a gentle, sustained inhalation.

Lie in the Relaxation Position (see pages 94–95). **Breathe in** gently through your nose, taking the breath in laterally, so that you gently fill the sides and back of your ribcage with air. As you start to **breathe out** slowly through your mouth, feel your stomach start to sink down towards the floor. As you **continue to breathe out**, allow your stomach to sink down a little further by gently drawing in your abdominal muscles and gathering in your waistline a little to stabilize, and to give your body some support. This is a very subtle movement that requires focus, but little effort. The exhalation does not cause your spine to move at all. Gently inhale through your nose, taking the air into the sides and back of your ribcage again. Then repeat the exhalation as above.

Repeat for 6–10 breaths

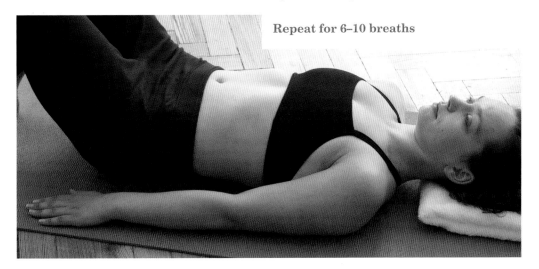

SHOULDER STABILIZATION

This is essential for creating a stable core. You need to be able to stabilize your shoulders correctly so that you are in good alignment and can move your arms to reach or lift freely. Poor shoulder stabilization frequently leads to stiff, painful shoulders, chronic neck pain and headaches. Improving your shoulder stabilization helps to reduce these problems by releasing tension in the neck and shoulders. It also strengthens the muscles that stabilize your shoulder blades, and teaches good head, neck and shoulder alignment.

As you exercise, particularly if you are finding a movement tricky to perform, you may find your shoulders are the first area to tense up. Suddenly, you are lifting your shoulders incorrectly and/or drawing your shoulder blades too far in together. To prevent this, you need to stabilize your shoulders by sliding your shoulder blades down into your back and then around, so that they wrap forwards slightly towards the sides of your ribcage. It helps to think of gliding the outer edges of your shoulder blades down, while spreading them wide across your back, so maintaining a feeling of width and openness across your collarbones. Try it for yourself, by slowly lifting one arm above your head, as shown first incorrectly, then correctly, in the photographs below – the aim is never to fix the shoulder blades down, but to allow them to glide down and around naturally.

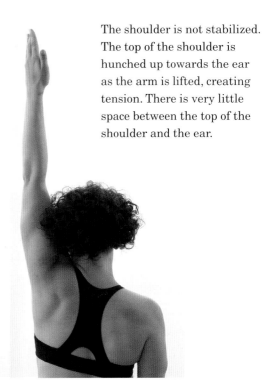

The shoulder is not stabilized. The top of the shoulder is hunched up towards the ear as the arm is lifted, creating tension. There is very little space between the top of the shoulder and the ear.

The shoulder has been gently stabilized by sliding the shoulder blade down into the back and gliding it around towards the side of the ribcage. The shoulder blades are spread wider apart, and there is much more space between the top of the shoulder and the ear.

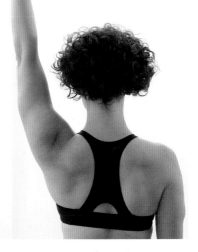

TEACHER'S TIP

• Throughout the exercises that follow, whenever you see the instruction 'stabilize your shoulders' or 'glide your shoulder blades down and around', it is this movement that is being described in shorthand.

Knee Fold

THIS EXERCISE TEACHES YOU HOW TO CENTRE
AND STABILIZE YOUR CORE. THROUGH
LATERAL BREATHING AND STABILIZING, YOU
WILL LEARN HOW TO PREVENT YOUR PELVIS
FROM ROCKING FORWARD OR BACKWARD, OR
SHIFTING TO ONE SIDE OR THE OTHER, AS YOU
RAISE YOUR LEG.

1 Lie in the Relaxation Position
(see pages 94–95). **Breathe in**
gently through your nose,
taking the air into the sides and back
of your ribcage.

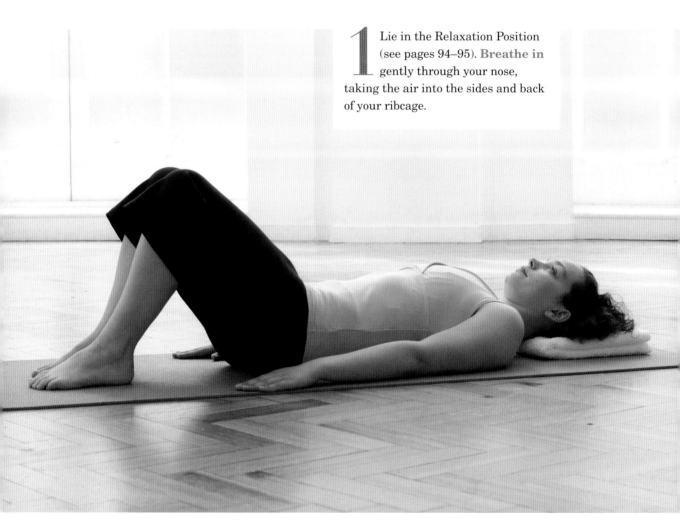

- Focus on keeping your lower abdominals, in particular, drawing in as you perform the exercise. Don't allow your stomach muscles to bulge outwards.
- Fold your knee in, without disturbing the alignment of your pelvis, or losing your neutral spine.

- Think of your thighbone dropping down into your hip socket as you fold your leg in.
- Don't allow your shoulders to hunch up, or your neck to arch. Keep your shoulders relaxed, and keep the back of your neck lengthened at all times.

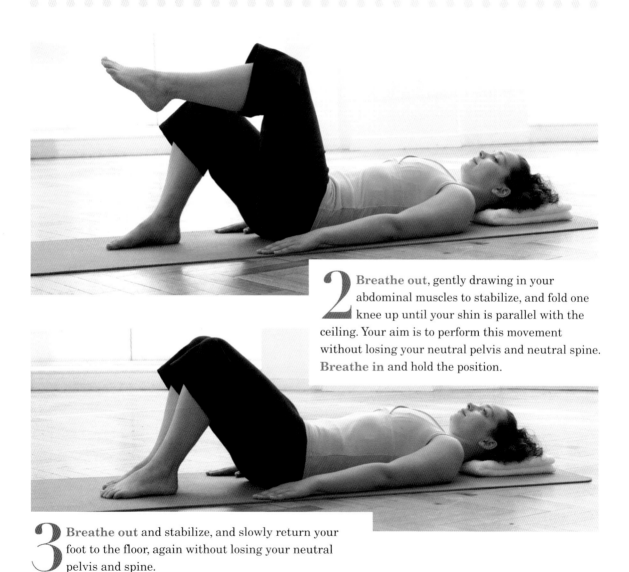

2 **Breathe out,** gently drawing in your abdominal muscles to stabilize, and fold one knee up until your shin is parallel with the ceiling. Your aim is to perform this movement without losing your neutral pelvis and neutral spine. **Breathe in** and hold the position.

3 **Breathe out** and stabilize, and slowly return your foot to the floor, again without losing your neutral pelvis and spine.

Repetitions: 5 Knee Folds on each leg, alternating legs

Arm Splits

THIS EXERCISE TEACHES YOU HOW TO
CONTROL YOUR RIBCAGE, SO THAT YOU
REMAIN IN NEUTRAL SPINE THROUGHOUT
THE EXERCISE. IT ENCOURAGES GOOD
SHOULDER STABILIZATION AND IMPROVES
SHOULDER MOBILITY.

1 Lie on your back in the Relaxation
Position (see pages 94–95). Reach
your arms up to the ceiling. You
should keep them straight without locking
your elbows, and with your palms facing
away from you. **Breathe in**.

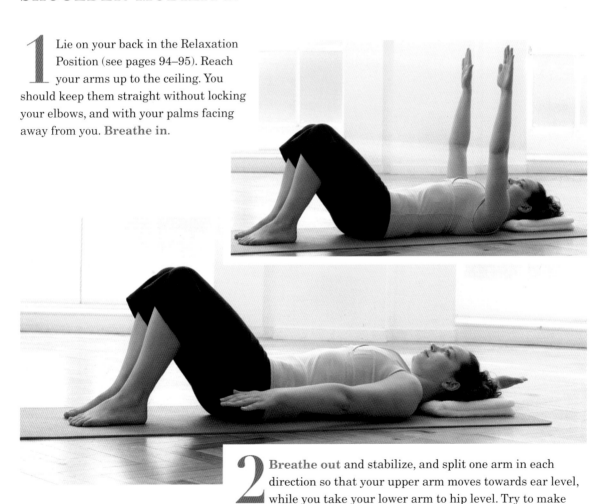

2 **Breathe out** and stabilize, and split one arm in each
direction so that your upper arm moves towards ear level,
while you take your lower arm to hip level. Try to make
this movement by gliding your shoulder blades down into your
back and then around towards the side of your ribcage, so that the
tops of your shoulders don't hunch up towards your ears.

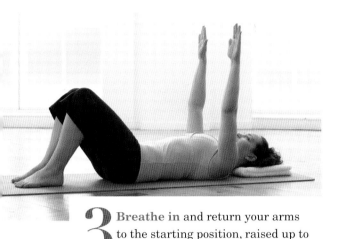

3 Breathe in and return your arms to the starting position, raised up to the ceiling.

TEACHER'S TIPS

- Remain in neutral pelvis and neutral spine throughout.

- Be careful not to arch your back and let your ribcage flare. It helps to think of keeping your ribcage connected to your spine.

- Only take your arm back as far as you can maintain stability in your shoulder. Aim for quality of movement, rather than trying to force your arm too low so that the top of your shoulder hunches up towards your ear, and your elbow bends.

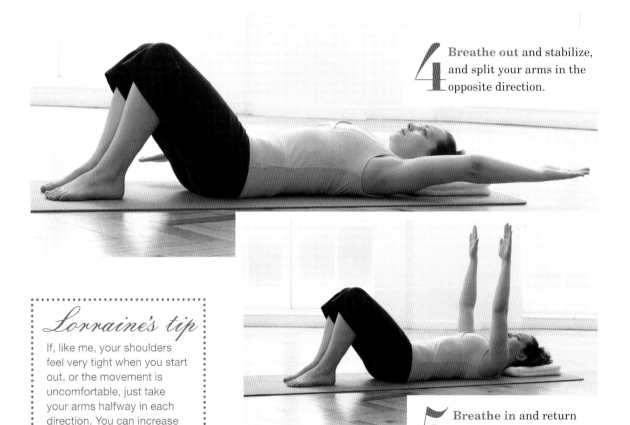

4 Breathe out and stabilize, and split your arms in the opposite direction.

Lorraine's tip

If, like me, your shoulders feel very tight when you start out, or the movement is uncomfortable, just take your arms halfway in each direction. You can increase the range of movement as you become more familiar with the exercise.

5 Breathe in and return your arms to the ceiling.

Repetitions: 6–10 Arm Splits on each side, alternating sides

Pelvic Curl

THIS EXERCISE FOCUSES ON CORE STABILITY,
STRENGTHENS YOUR ABDOMINAL MUSCLES
AND IMPROVES YOUR SPINAL MOBILITY
AND FLEXIBILITY.

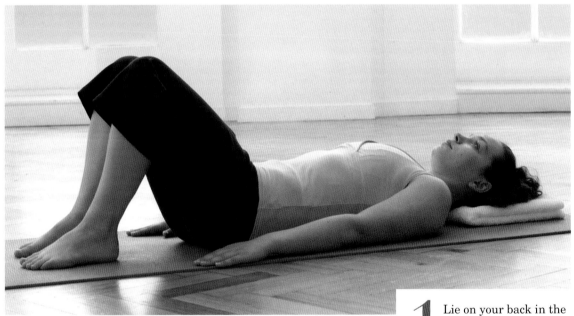

1 Lie on your back in the Relaxation Position (see pages 94–95). **Breathe in**, gently inhaling through your nose, taking the air into the sides and back of your ribcage.

TEACHER'S TIPS

- Feel that you are using your abdominal muscles to curl up and down.
- Watch that your knees don't fall any further apart.
- Be careful not to tense your neck or hunch your shoulders. Slide your shoulder blades down into your back and around towards the sides of your ribcage, and keep the back of your neck lengthened.
- Try to isolate the vertebrae in your spine more, each time you repeat the exercise.
- Be careful not to thrust your ribs forward or arch your back.

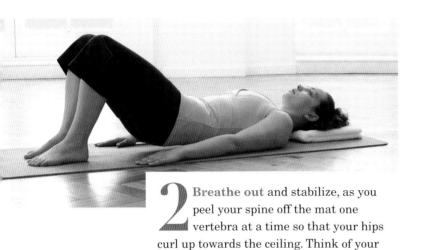

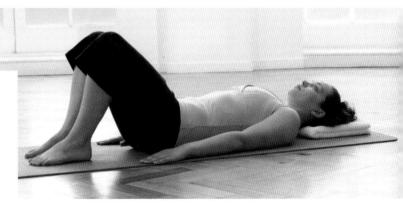

Lorraine's tip

If this exercise feels tough, or you feel any tension in your back, shoulders or neck, try coming up halfway, or even less than that, until you become more able to perform the movement. This worked for me.

2 **Breathe out** and stabilize, as you peel your spine off the mat one vertebra at a time so that your hips curl up towards the ceiling. Think of your knees moving forward over your toes as you curl up.

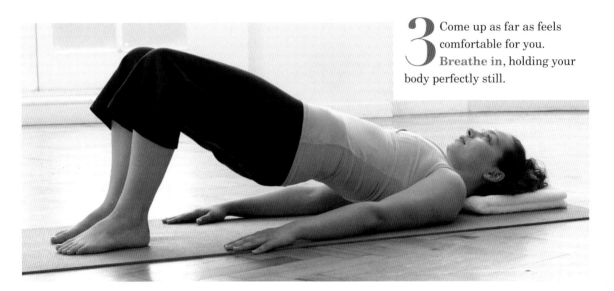

3 Come up as far as feels comfortable for you. **Breathe in**, holding your body perfectly still.

4 **Breathe out** and stabilize, and slowly roll down through your spine, lowering one vertebra at a time. Imagine your spine is melting into the mat as you peel down.

Repetitions: 6–10 Pelvic Curls

Hip Roll

THIS EXERCISE TRIMS YOUR WAISTLINE. IT ALSO
IMPROVES SPINAL MOBILITY AS YOUR SPINE
GENTLY ROTATES FROM SIDE TO SIDE, AND
HELPS TO RELEASE TENSION IN THE BACK.

1 Lie in the Relaxation Position (see pages 94–95). Bring your knees and feet together. Take your arms out to the sides into a T position, with palms facing the floor. Squeeze your inner thighs together and keep this gentle connection throughout, so that your knees and feet remain together during the exercise. **Breathe in**.

2 **Breathe out** and stabilize, and carefully roll your knees over to one side, while keeping both shoulder blades flat on the mat. Turn your head gently to the opposite side. Your feet should roll along with your knees, but one foot should remain in contact with the mat. **Breathe in**, holding this position.

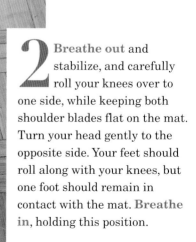

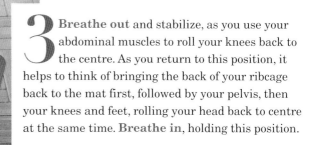

3 Breathe out and stabilize, as you use your abdominal muscles to roll your knees back to the centre. As you return to this position, it helps to think of bringing the back of your ribcage back to the mat first, followed by your pelvis, then your knees and feet, rolling your head back to centre at the same time. **Breathe in**, holding this position.

4 Breathe out and stabilize, and roll your knees over to the opposite side this time, turning your head gently in the other direction. **Breathe in**, holding this position.

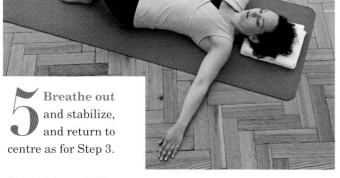

5 Breathe out and stabilize, and return to centre as for Step 3.

Repetitions: 5 Hip Rolls on each side, alternating sides

TEACHER'S TIPS

• Ensure that you roll over carefully, without twisting your hips out of alignment or allowing your ribs to flare.

• Only roll a small distance, and make sure that you feel entirely comfortable throughout.

• Relax your neck and chest, and maintain your shoulder stabilization.

Chest Curl

THIS EXERCISE STRENGTHENS THE
ABDOMINAL MUSCLES FOR A FIRMER,
FLATTER STOMACH. IT ALSO HELPS TO
IMPROVE YOUR SPINAL FLEXIBILITY AND
CHALLENGES YOU TO REMAIN IN NEUTRAL
PELVIS, WITH GOOD CORE STABILIZATION.

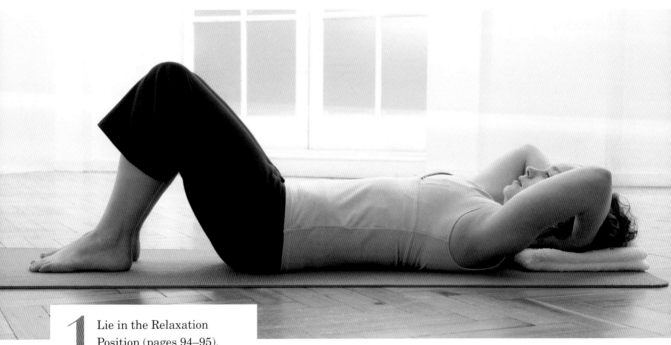

1 Lie in the Relaxation
Position (pages 94–95).
Take your hands behind
your head, interlacing your fingers
to cradle and support your head.
Open your elbows out to the side,
so that you can just see them
within your peripheral vision. Feel
the weight of your head within
your hands. **Breathe in.**

Lorraine's tip
You might find that you can't maintain
a neutral pelvis and that you tuck your
pelvis under as you curl forward, pressing
your lower back into the mat. If this is
the case, try it again without coming up
so high.

- To curl off the mat, think of sliding your ribcage along the front of your body towards your hips, keeping the front of your body flat and long throughout.
- Continue to draw in your abdominal muscles as you curl forwards. Watch that your lower abdominal muscles do not bulge outwards as you curl.

- Keep your head heavy in your hands throughout, and ensure that you are curling forwards with your abdominal muscles, rather than using your neck muscles to lift your head. Keep the back of your neck lengthened at all times.
- Maintain a neutral pelvis at all times, so that your pelvis doesn't tuck under or overarch.

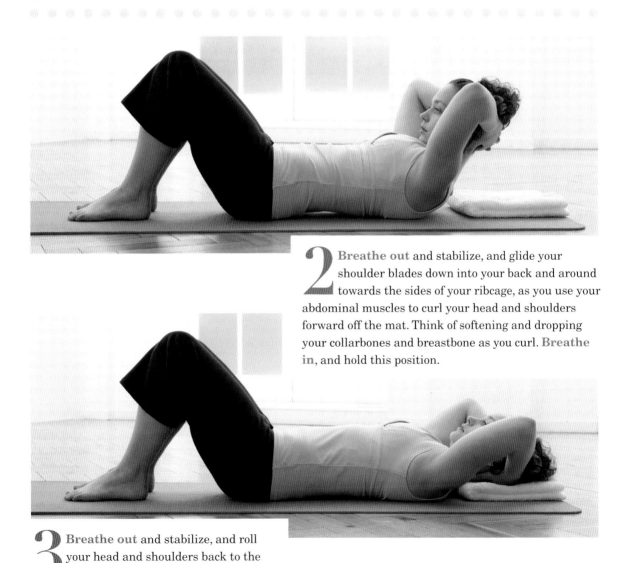

2 Breathe out and stabilize, and glide your shoulder blades down into your back and around towards the sides of your ribcage, as you use your abdominal muscles to curl your head and shoulders forward off the mat. Think of softening and dropping your collarbones and breastbone as you curl. Breathe in, and hold this position.

3 Breathe out and stabilize, and roll your head and shoulders back to the mat with control.

Repetitions: 6–10 Chest Curls

Oblique Curl

THIS EXERCISE IMPROVES YOUR CORE
STABILITY, STRENGTHENS YOUR ABDOMINAL
MUSCLES AND WHITTLES YOUR WAISTLINE.
IT ALSO IMPROVES YOUR SPINAL
FLEXIBILITY AND MOBILITY.

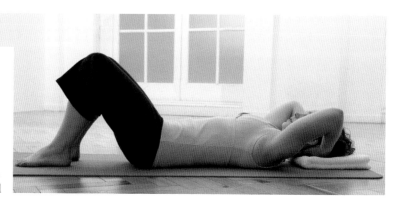

1 Lie in the Relaxation Position (see pages 94–95). Take your hands behind your head, interlacing your fingers to cradle and support your head. Open your elbows out to the side, so that you can just see them within your peripheral vision. Feel the weight of your head within your hands. **Breathe in**.

2 **Breathe out** and stabilize, and glide your shoulder blades down into your back and around towards the sides of your ribcage, as you use your abdominal muscles to curl your head and shoulders forward off the mat. Think of softening and dropping your collarbones and breastbone as you curl. (You are now in Step 2 of the Chest Curl, see page 107). **Breathe in**, and hold this position.

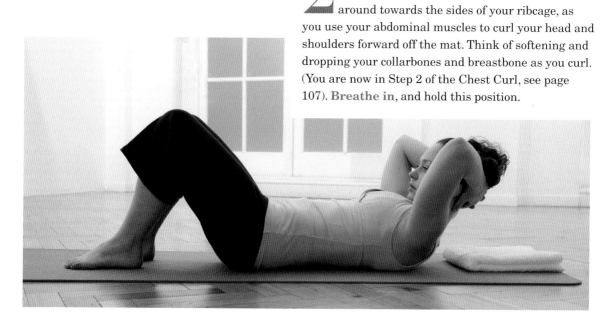

- Maintain your neutral pelvic position at all times. In particular, don't let your pelvis tuck under as you curl forward.
- Keep your head heavy in your hands.
- Do not side bend as you curl. To prevent this, keep the length on both sides of your waist.
- Don't allow your shoulders to hunch up towards your ears; maintain your shoulder stability at all times.

3 Breathe out, rotating your lower ribcage very slightly to one side, as you continue to stabilize your shoulders, keeping your shoulder blades wide across your back, and your collarbones wide and open. This small rotation comes from the ribcage, and not by twisting your shoulders. Your elbows should remain the same distance apart at all times.

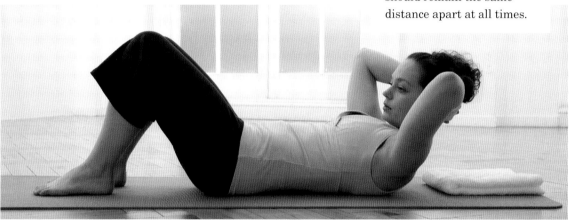

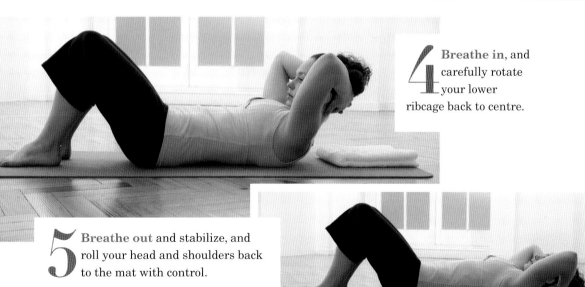

4 Breathe in, and carefully rotate your lower ribcage back to centre.

5 Breathe out and stabilize, and roll your head and shoulders back to the mat with control.

Repetitions: 5 Oblique Curls on each side, alternating sides

Table Top

THIS TEACHES YOU HOW TO STABILIZE AND
SUPPORT YOUR BODY, AND HELPS TO IMPROVE
YOUR ALIGNMENT. YOU WILL NEED TO GIVE
THIS EXERCISE YOUR FULL CONCENTRATION IF
YOU ARE TO PERFORM IT WELL – IT IS MORE
CHALLENGING THAN IT FIRST APPEARS.

1 Kneel on all fours, with your hands directly under your shoulders, and your knees directly under your hips. Your feet should be in line with your knees. Your gaze is directly down at the floor, with the back of your neck lengthened. **Breathe in**.

2 **Breathe out** and stabilize, and slide one leg away from you along the floor in line with your hip, keeping your toes in contact with the floor. At the same time, slide your opposite arm along the floor, in line with your shoulder, keeping your fingers in contact with the mat. Your aim is to make this movement whilst stabilizing your centre, so that your trunk remains perfectly still like a table top throughout, without losing the alignment of your pelvis.

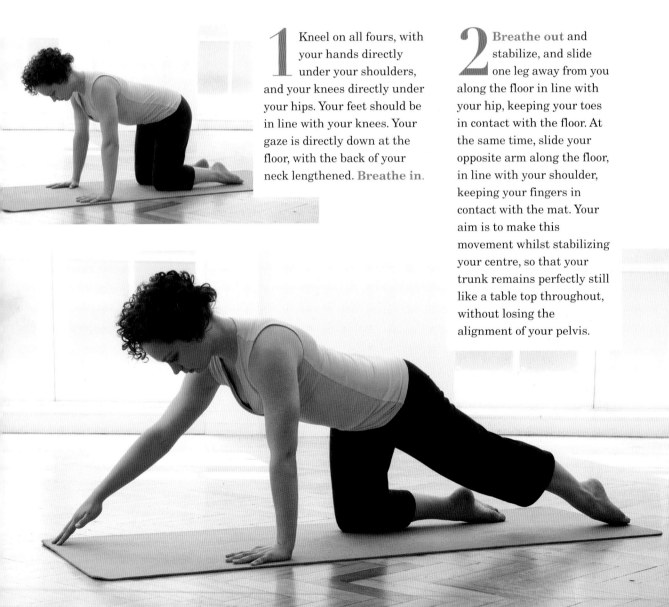

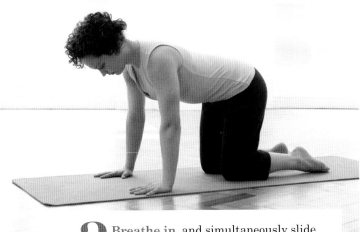

3 Breathe in, and simultaneously slide your leg and arm back in, again trying to keep your trunk completely still.

Repetitions: 5 Table Tops on each side, alternating sides

TEACHER'S TIP

- Maintain your shoulder stability at all times.
- Don't allow your pelvis to become unbalanced so that one of your hips drops forward, or hikes up.
- Apart from your moving leg and arm, your aim is to keep the rest of your body perfectly still.
- Watch that you don't rotate your thigh inwards or outwards within your hip socket as you move.

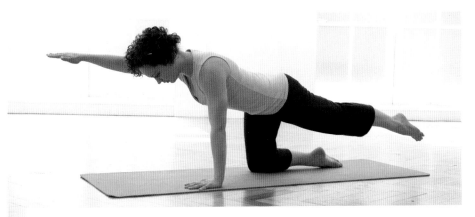

VARIATION

Once you can perform the above exercise well, you can challenge your core stability further whilst toning your buttocks.

Follow Steps 1–2 of the exercise above. **Breathe in** and remain perfectly still with one leg and the opposite arm outstretched, with your hand and foot still in contact with the mat. **Breathe out** and stabilize, and simultaneously lift your arm and leg no higher than your body, stabilizing

your shoulders as you move. Your leg stays in line with your hip, your arm with your shoulder. Your pelvis remains square to the floor, so that your back remains like a table top throughout. **Breathe in**, lowering both limbs to the mat, and then **Breathe out**, sliding both limbs back in, without losing alignment.

Repetitions: 5 modified Table Tops on each side, alternating sides

Clam

THIS CHALLENGES YOUR CORE STABILITY
AND STRENGTHENS BUTTOCK MUSCLES. THIS
EXERCISE AND THE ONE THAT FOLLOWS FLOW
TOGETHER BETTER IF YOU PERFORM EACH ON
ONE SIDE FIRST, BEFORE REPEATING BOTH
EXERCISES ON THE OTHER SIDE.

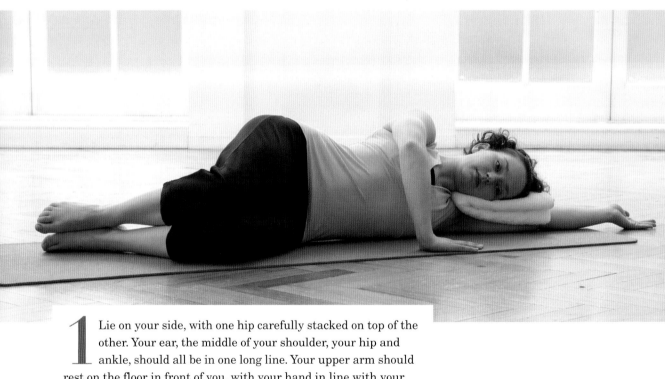

1 Lie on your side, with one hip carefully stacked on top of the other. Your ear, the middle of your shoulder, your hip and ankle, should all be in one long line. Your upper arm should rest on the floor in front of you, with your hand in line with your shoulder, for support. Your lower arm should stretch out above your head, palm up. You may place a folded towel or pillow between your head and your arm, so that your neck is in line with your spine. If you find it difficult to know if you are in a straight line or not, try lining your body up with the edge of the mat. Now, slide both knees forward, without changing the rest of your alignment, until your heels are in line with your bottom. **Breathe in.**

- Think of rotating your thigh bone into your hip socket as the knee opens.
- Your upper body should remain still and relaxed. Watch that you don't hunch your shoulders or round them forward.

- Don't collapse your waist into the mat. Maintain your core stability. You should be able to slip a hand in the space between your waist and the mat, as your leg opens.
- As you open your leg, keep your feet together at all times.

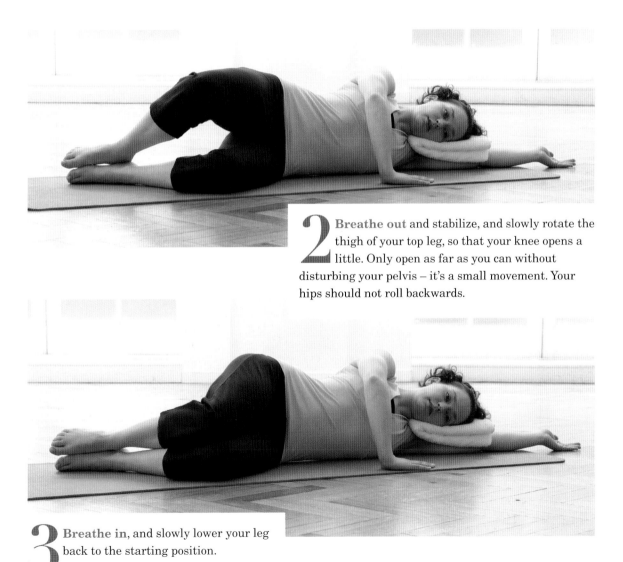

2 **Breathe out** and stabilize, and slowly rotate the thigh of your top leg, so that your knee opens a little. Only open as far as you can without disturbing your pelvis – it's a small movement. Your hips should not roll backwards.

3 **Breathe in**, and slowly lower your leg back to the starting position.

Repetitions: 6–10 Clams on each side

Torpedo

THIS EXERCISE CHALLENGES YOUR CORE
STABILITY, TRIMS YOUR WAISTLINE AND
STRENGTHENS YOUR THIGHS.

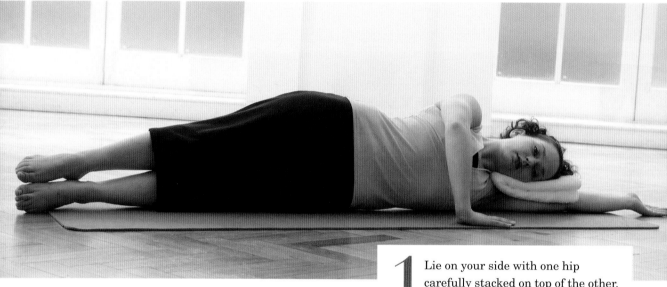

TEACHER'S TIPS

• Make sure your legs don't swing behind you as
you lift.

• It's very important that you keep the space
between your waist and the mat as you lift.

• As you lift or lower your leg, lengthen through
your whole body. Keep your waistline long and
reach out your legs.

• Your hand is in front of you for gentle support. Try
not to grip on to the floor for dear life. The more
you stabilize from your centre, the less you will
need your hand to support you.

• Keep your elbow open and your shoulders
stabilized throughout.

1 Lie on your side with one hip
carefully stacked on top of the other.
Your ear, the middle of your shoulder
and your hip and ankle should all be in one
long line. Your upper arm should rest on
the floor in front of you, with your hand in
line with your shoulder, for support. Your
lower arm should stretch out above your
head, palm up. You may place a folded
towel or pillow between your head and
your arm, so that your neck is in line with
your spine. If you find it difficult to know if
you are in a straight line or not, try lining
your body up with the edge of the mat.
Breathe in.

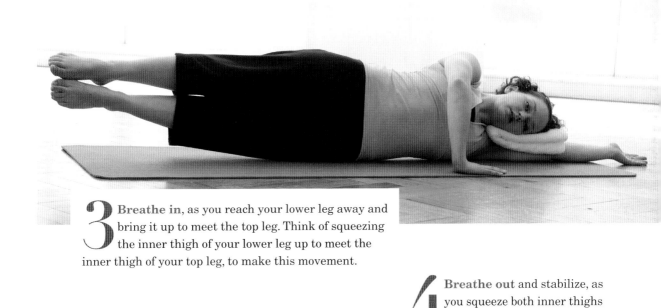

2 Breathe out and stabilize, and lift your top leg to hip height, without tipping your pelvis. Imagine you are trying to stretch your leg away from your torso as you move.

Lorraine's tip

I found this very challenging at first, and could not perform the exercise without rolling my hips and losing stability. If you find that's the case too, try this Pilates modification: Do Steps 1–2 only – lifting just the top leg – until you feel confident enough to tackle the exercise in full.

3 Breathe in, as you reach your lower leg away and bring it up to meet the top leg. Think of squeezing the inner thigh of your lower leg up to meet the inner thigh of your top leg, to make this movement.

4 Breathe out and stabilize, as you squeeze both inner thighs together and reach your legs away as you lower them to the starting position.

Repetitions: 6–10 Torpedoes on each side

Diamond Press

THIS EXERCISE TEACHES YOU TO STABILIZE
YOUR CORE WHEN LYING ON YOUR FRONT. IT
ALSO GENTLY EXTENDS (BACKWARD BENDS)
YOUR SPINE TO IMPROVE MOBILITY, AND
STRENGTHENS YOUR UPPER BACK MUSCLES.

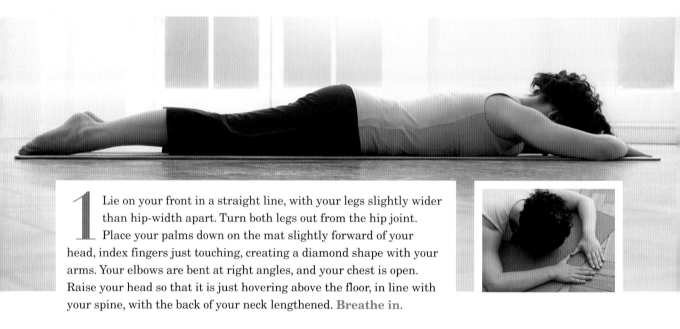

1 Lie on your front in a straight line, with your legs slightly wider than hip-width apart. Turn both legs out from the hip joint. Place your palms down on the mat slightly forward of your head, index fingers just touching, creating a diamond shape with your arms. Your elbows are bent at right angles, and your chest is open. Raise your head so that it is just hovering above the floor, in line with your spine, with the back of your neck lengthened. **Breathe in.**

TEACHER'S TIPS

- Don't let your head tip backwards. Continue to look down at the mat throughout the exercise, with the back of your neck lengthened.

- Allow both the crown of your head and your chest to lengthen forward as you lift.

- The bottom of your ribcage should stay in contact with the mat at all times.

- Keep stabilizing your core, so that your abdominal muscles lift away from the mat as you lift.

- If you feel an ache or pinching in your lower back as you lift, stop immediately. Repeat the exercise again, whilst trying to stabilize your core more and don't come up quite so high. You could also try slipping a folded towel or pillow under your hips to support your lower back. If you still feel a pinch, leave this exercise out for now, and return to it when your core stability has improved.

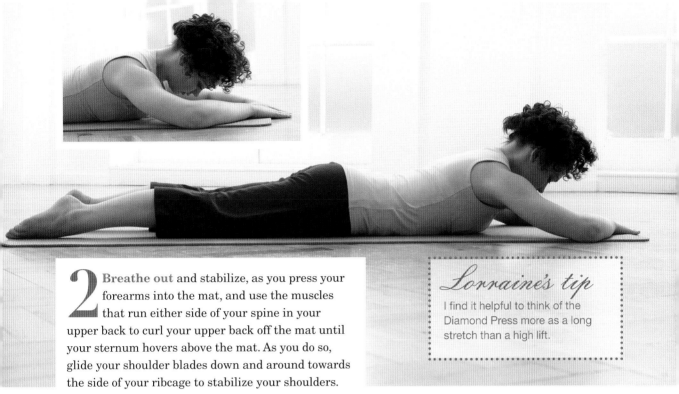

2 Breathe out and stabilize, as you press your forearms into the mat, and use the muscles that run either side of your spine in your upper back to curl your upper back off the mat until your sternum hovers above the mat. As you do so, glide your shoulder blades down and around towards the side of your ribcage to stabilize your shoulders.

Lorraine's tip

I find it helpful to think of the Diamond Press more as a long stretch than a high lift.

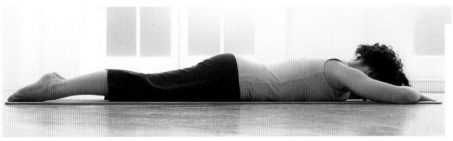

3 Breathe in, as you lower down with control.

Repetitions: 6–10 Diamond Presses

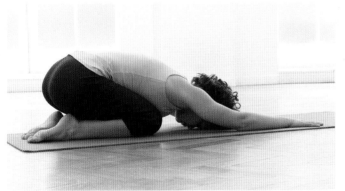

REST POSITION

After performing the Diamond Press, end in the Rest Position. It's a great opportunity to cool down at the end of your session, and stretches your spine beautifully.

From the Diamond Press position, draw your body back so that you are sitting on your heels with your arms stretched out in front of you. Rest here for approximately 30 seconds. Slowly roll back up to a kneeling position, one vertebra at a time to finish.

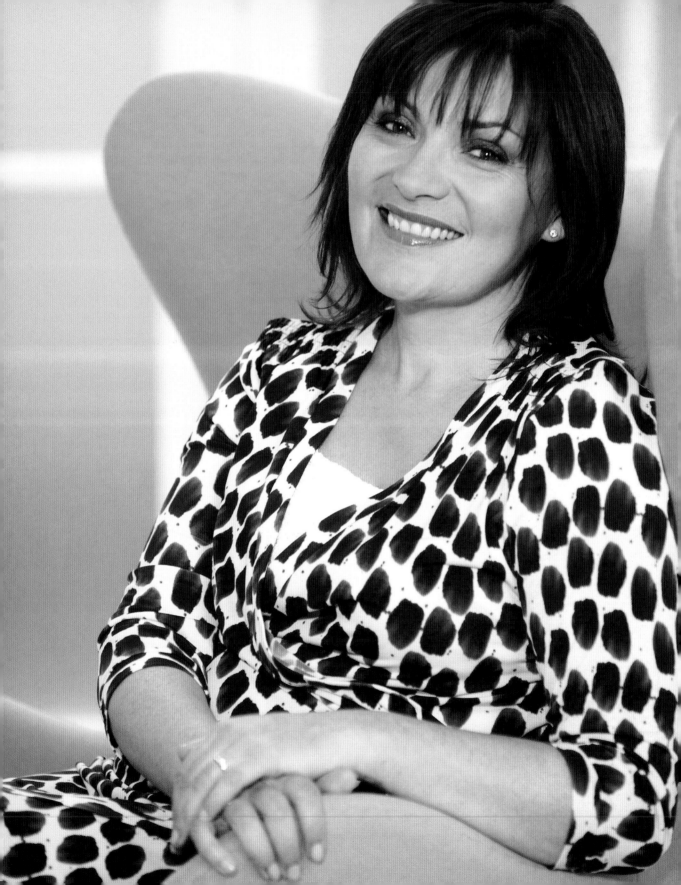

LOOKING GREAT

Looking younger

I HAVE BEEN LUCKY ENOUGH TO INHERIT MY MUM'S HIGH CHEEKBONES AND GOOD SKIN AND, BECAUSE I HAVE NEVER SMOKED AND TAKE CARE TO KEEP MY FACE OUT OF THE SUNSHINE, I LOOK – IN THE WORDS OF EAMONN HOLMES – 'NOT TOO BAD FOR AN AULD BIRD'.

I was immensely cheered by the revelation from Kim Cattrall, who plays Samantha in *Sex and the City* and looks stunning at 50+, that she 'literally works her ass off'. Kim watches what she eats, rarely drinks alcohol and goes through a punishing daily exercise regime. While all of her hard work has undoubtedly paid off, most of us simply don't have the time, money or willpower to look that stunning. However, there are lots of things you can do to look younger without having to take on such a brutal regime or succumbing to plastic surgery.

THE SECRETS OF YOUTH

Looking younger than you are has a bit to do with luck, but is mostly about lifestyle, and it is never too late to make changes.

Quit smoking It gives you deep wrinkles and gives your skin a tired, grey pallor.

Drink plenty of water Make sure you drink at least 6–8 glasses of water a day to keep your skin hydrated and to plump up fine lines.

Enjoy alcohol in moderation Too much booze takes its toll on your face, causing dehydration, wrinkles and broken veins, so don't overdo it.

LOOKING YOUNGER THAN YOU ARE HAS A BIT TO DO WITH LUCK, BUT IT IS MOSTLY ABOUT LIFESTYLE, AND IT IS NEVER TOO LATE TO MAKE CHANGES

Stay out of the sun Joan Collins has never exposed her face to the rays of the sun. She wears factor 60 sun block and a large, floppy hat and, as a result, she has the skin of a woman half her age. There's more on sun safety on pages 122–23.

Stress less Being tense makes you hunch up your body and frown, both guaranteed to make you look older. Try to make time to relax and unwind each day.

Moisturize night and day As we age, our skin loses its resilience and becomes thinner and drier, so it's important to remember to moisturize regularly twice a day.

Stay in shape A toned, supple body will make you feel and look younger and regular exercise is absolutely vital for keeping your bones and muscles strong.

Eat the right food If you eat badly, it will show in your face and in your figure: your muscles won't be strong and your skin will sag. If you want to look younger, take a good, hard look at your everyday diet and make what changes you need to. (See Chapter 1: Healthy Eating)

Think young If you want to look young, you need to think young. A recent US study has shown that

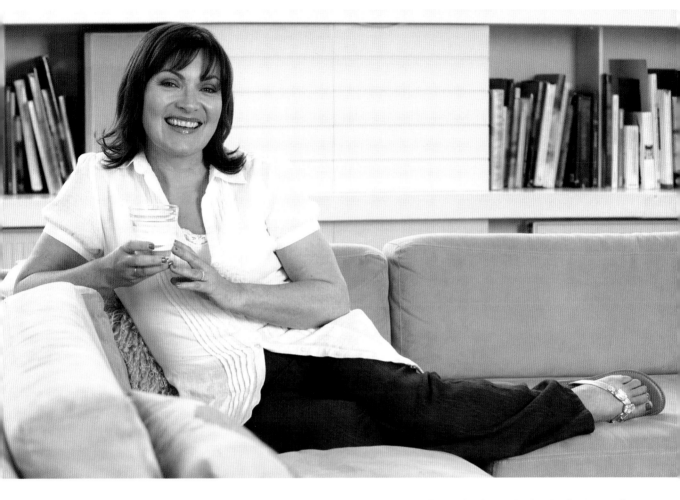

people with an upbeat view of life age slower. Being open to new ideas and trends, really enjoying life and having fun will make you look and feel more youthful.

KEEP SMILING

As a last piece of advice, I really believe that you should smile more! I always think that our faces reflect our personalities and that when we get older we have the faces we deserve. So, if you have been mostly miserable, it will show in the droop of your eyes, the downward curve of your mouth and the wrinkles of bad temper. If you have a sunny disposition, you will still have lines – but they will be laughter lines and you will appear younger, happier and more attractive.

QUICK FIXES TO LOOK YOUNGER

- Get a good night's sleep
- Watch that posture – stand up straight
- Get a new haircut with lowlights or highlights
- Whiten your teeth
- Change your make-up
- Moisturize, moisturize, moisturize
- Keep active
- Start Pilates classes
- Take up a hobby
- Make new friends
- Smile!

Your skin and sun

WHEN I WAS IN MY TWENTIES, I USED TO GO ON HOLIDAY AND LIE IN THE SUN FOR HOURS. I'M LUCKY I DIDN'T CAUSE LONG-TERM DAMAGE TO MY SKIN. SINCE MY THIRTIES I HAVE SLATHERED ON THE SUN BLOCK, POPPED ON A WIDE-BRIMMED HAT AND STAYED IN THE SHADE WHEN THE SUN IS AT ITS HOTTEST.

most people love sunshine, particularly here in the UK, where we often don't get as much as we'd like! And some sun is good for you. It helps form vitamin D, which is vital for strong bones, while a lack of sunshine can trigger SAD (seasonal affective disorder), which is a form of depression. However, exposing yourself to too much sun can have very serious consequences.

WHAT YOU NEED TO KNOW

As much as 80 per cent of skin damage – wrinkles, age spots, freckles, leathery skin texture and spider veins – is caused by the sun. It's a sobering thought that 80 per cent of what makes you look older could be prevented if you protect yourself properly from the sun. And it's never too late to begin – start now and you can limit the damage.

Sunburn is a true burn, just like a burn from boiling water. It causes tissue destruction, and repeatedly allowing your skin to burn increases the risk of developing skin cancer.

The vast majority of skin cancer cases are caused by exposure to ultraviolet (UV) rays from sunshine and sun beds, and are preventable. There are two kinds: non-melanoma skin cancer, which is the less serious form, and the potentially deadly

FAKE TAN – GOOD IDEA?

Yes. The only safe tan is a fake one. There are many products around that will give you a natural-looking sun-kissed glow as long as you apply them properly. Here's how:

1 Start by exfoliating – this is vital for a streak-free tan and will make colour go on more smoothly. Pay particular attention to places like knees and elbows, where the skin tends to be tougher and more wrinkled.

2 Dry yourself and apply body lotion. You need to leave at least 30 minutes for this to sink in thoroughly before applying the fake tan.

3 Apply your fake tan by working in small areas at a time. Use even, circular motions – not up and down – with the flat of your hands. Apply sparingly to hands and feet and try to glide over spots like elbows where the fake tan tends to accumulate.

4 Don't overdo it – its better to build up gradually to get the right effect. Remember, you want to look sun-kissed, not like a satsuma!

5 When you're done wash your hands immediately to avoid staining. Don't forget to scrub between your fingers and under your nails.

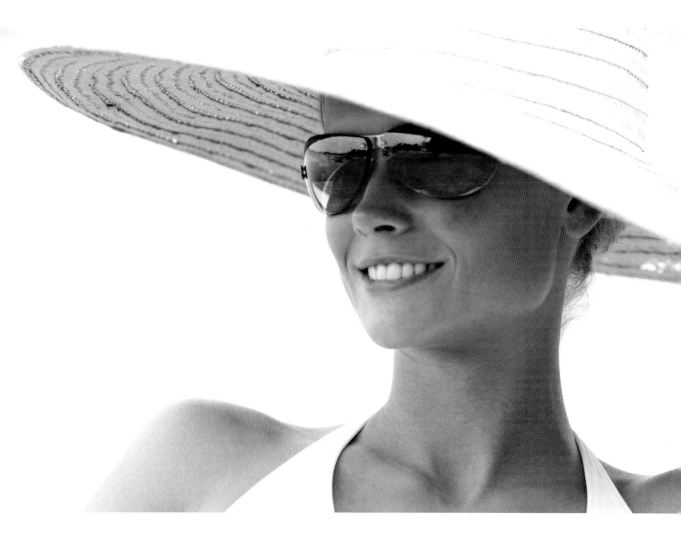

melanoma. Worryingly, the number of people in the UK diagnosed with melanoma has increased dramatically in the UK in recent years. We should all be more aware of the very real risks we are subjecting ourselves to by overexposure to the sun.

If you notice any changes to moles or skin pigmentation you should always see your doctor, particularly if you are fair-skinned.

HOW TO PROTECT YOURSELF

Always – every single day, even in winter – wear a sun block with a sun protection factor (SPF) of at least 15 on your face, hands and other exposed parts of your body. If you're skiing or on water, where UV rays are intensified, you should go for an SPF of 20–30.

Stay out of the sun between 11 am and 3 pm, when the sun's rays are at their most intense. Beware of hidden sun. Experts say that it's the 10–20 minutes of unprotected sun exposure – popping out to buy a sandwich at lunchtime or hanging out the washing, for instance – that do the most damage to skin over the years.

Cover up for maximum protection. Wear a wide-brimmed hat and opt for long sleeves and full-length trousers in cool fabrics when you're on holiday in the sun. Protect your eyes with sunglasses whenever you're outside in sunlight.

And finally: don't ever use sun beds.

Caring for your face

IF YOU PUT IN THE EFFORT WITH SKIN CARE
YOU WILL LOOK YOUNGER AND FEEL BETTER.
THERE'S NO POINT HAVING NUMEROUS
LOTIONS AND POTIONS SITTING ON THE
DRESSING TABLE AND THEN EXPECTING
THEM TO WORK BY MAGIC. YOU NEED TO
ACTUALLY USE THEM REGULARLY.

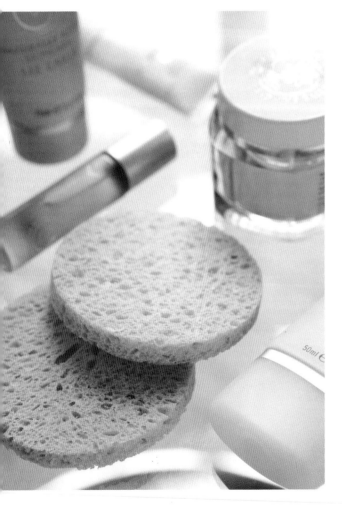

KNOW YOUR SKIN TYPE

To choose products that suit you and deliver
results you need to know what type of skin
you have:

- **Normal** Neither too oily or too dry, normal skin
  has no obvious problems.
- **Dry** Dry skin produces low levels of sebum and
  is often thin and rather translucent. It can be
  flaky in places.
- **Oily** This type of skin is often shiny because
  it produces excessive sebum, especially in the
  T-zone made up of your forehead, nose and chin.
- **Combination** Very common, this combines an
  oily central T-zone and a dryer, finer-skinned
  cheek area.
- **Sensitive** Delicate and easily irritated, sensitive
  skin reacts to things like cold weather and
  perfumed ingredients.

BEAUTY BASICS

Regardless of your skin type, these are the skin-
care essentials that you should have in your
bathroom cabinet.:

Cleanser To be healthy your skin needs to be
clean. There are cleansers for all types of skin and
all budgets, including wash-off and cream types.
A creamy cleanser tends to be the best choice for
more mature skin. Cleansing wipes are fine for

when you're travelling but they shouldn't replace a good routine.

Toner More astringent than cleanser, toner closes your pores as it removes make-up and dirt, leaving your skin feeling clean and refreshed. As always, be sure to choose a toner that's right for your skin type.

Moisturizer If you do just one thing for your face, moisturize it twice a day. Moisturizer generally comes in two versions: day cream and night cream. For the daytime always choose a moisturizer with a minimum SPF of 15. Night creams are richer and designed to feed your skin while you sleep. Your skin needs to breathe, though, so don't use one that is too rich or thick.

Eye cream or gel These are aimed at caring for the delicate skin around your eyes, which is 40 per cent finer than the rest of your skin.

Face mask Used once a week, this is a fantastic way to tone your skin and make it glow – not to mention a good excuse for spending some time relaxing in the bath.

Exfoliator One of the most effective ways to perk up your complexion is gently to slough off dead skin cells and reveal new, smooth cells with an facial exfoliator or polish. Exfoliating also reduces the appearance of fine wrinkles. Avoid the harsh ones that contain large particles and aim to use once or twice a week.

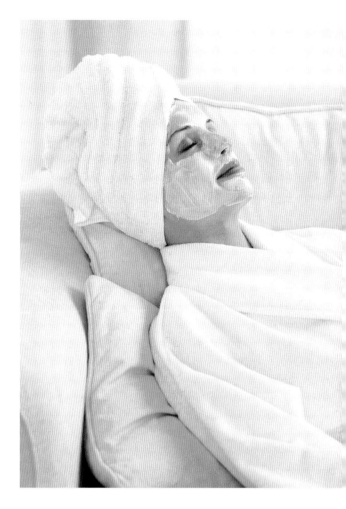

UNDERSTANDING LOTIONS AND POTIONS

Thousands of new skin-care products are launched each year, all promising that 'miracle ingredient' to make us look younger. No wonder we're confused! To help, here's a brief look at what's in many anti-ageing skin creams.

Alpha-hydroxy acids (AHAs) These encourage the skin to shed dead surface cells and plump up the skin to give a more youthful appearance. They are found naturally in unripe fruit and milk and they're not a new discovery – legendary beauty, Cleopatra, is renowned for having bathed in milk to protect her skin.

Beta-hydroxy acids (BHAs) These reduce the appearance of wrinkles and can even out patchy pigmentation. They're less abrasive than AHAs, which makes them much more suitable for sensitive skins.

Retinoids These anti-ageing ingredients are derived from vitamin A and help rejuvenate the skin by encouraging the formation of collagen and elastin, which tend to become depleted as we get older, making our skin sag. Retinoids give skin a smoother, more plumped-up appearance.

Antioxidants These ingredients combat the damage that free radicals – chemicals that attack cells – do to the collagen in our skin as we age. This damage causes visible signs of ageing on the face. Three powerful antioxidants found in skin-care products are vitamins A, C and E.

My skincare routine

I HAVE TO WEAR SO MUCH MAKE-UP FOR
TV THAT, ON THE DAYS WHEN I AM FILMING,
I REALLY NEED AN EXTRA-SPECIAL
CLEANSING ROUTINE. I USE A CLEANSING
CREAM WITH A WARM, MOIST MUSLIN
CLOTH, WHICH GETS OFF EVERY SINGLE
TRACE OF FOUNDATION AND MASCARA.

MY DAILY ROUTINE

This is the basic skin-care routine that I follow every night. In the mornings I repeat the routine, leaving out steps 4 and 5. You only need to cleanse once in the morning, but should cleanse twice in the evening to ensure that you have removed every bit of grease and make-up. No matter how tired you feel, you should never go to bed with make-up on.

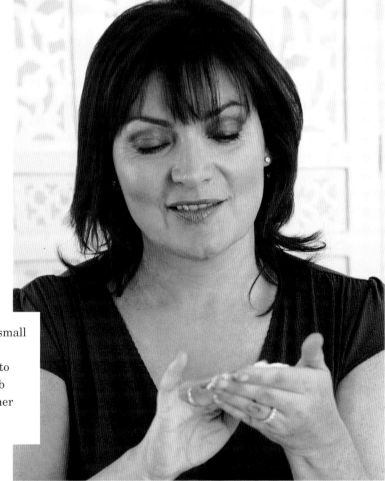

1 Squeeze a small amount of cleanser into your palm and rub your hands together to create a lather.

2 Use your fingers to apply the cleanser in small circular motions. You should start on your upper chest, below your collarbone and work your way upwards, making sure you cover your throat, chin, cheeks, nose and forehead. You should always work in this order, from chest to forehead, in order to avoid dragging the skin downwards.

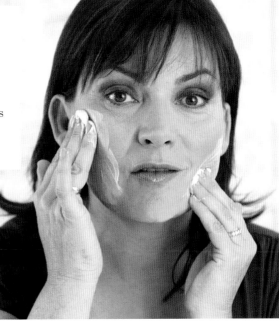

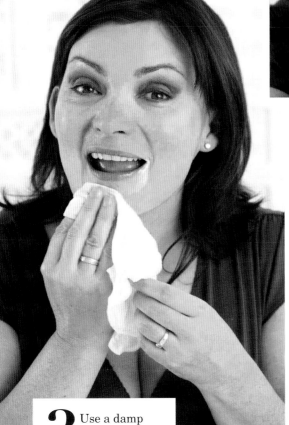

3 Use a damp muslin cloth to remove all the cleanser from your skin.

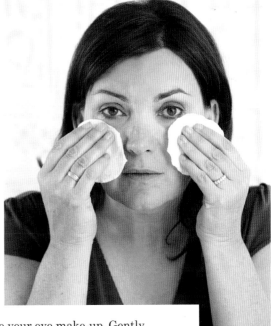

4 Next, remove your eye make-up. Gently massage some cleanser around the eye area using the tips of your fingers and working in tiny circles. Then gently remove the cleanser from around your eyes using cotton pads.

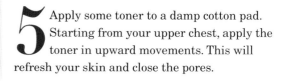

5 Apply some toner to a damp cotton pad. Starting from your upper chest, apply the toner in upward movements. This will refresh your skin and close the pores.

6 You can keep your eye-lifting gel in the refrigerator to make this step feel extra refreshing. Squeeze a dot of eye-lifting gel, about the size of a grain of rice, on to the tip of your ring finger. Touch the tip of your ring finger with the ring finger of your other hand, so that you have equal amounts of gel on both fingers.

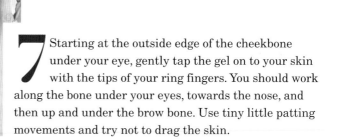

7 Starting at the outside edge of the cheekbone under your eye, gently tap the gel on to your skin with the tips of your ring fingers. You should work along the bone under your eyes, towards the nose, and then up and under the brow bone. Use tiny little patting movements and try not to drag the skin.

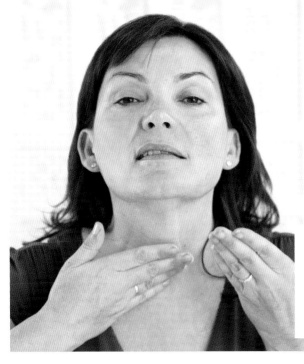

I ALWAYS USE TONER AND THEN APPLY PLENTY OF EYE CREAM AND MOISTURIZER.

8 Squeeze a small amount of moisturizer into your palm and rub your hands together. Starting at your upper chest and working upwards, gently massage the moisturizer into your skin.

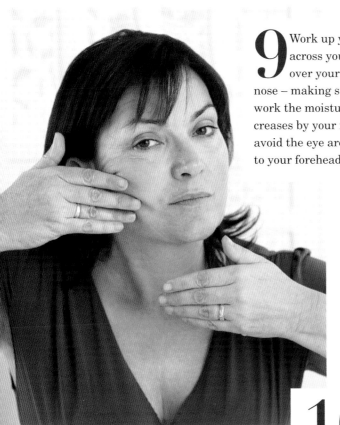

9 Work up your neck, across your chin and over your cheeks and nose – making sure that you work the moisturizer into the creases by your nose and avoid the eye area – and up to your forehead.

10 Finally, moisturize the back of your neck.

Essential hand care

IF THERE IS ONE PART OF YOUR BODY THAT
REALLY GIVES AWAY YOUR AGE IT HAS TO
BE THE HANDS. OUR HANDS TAKE A LOT OF
PUNISHMENT AND WE NEED TO LOOK AFTER
THEM. HAVING A ROUTINE OF BASIC HAND
CARE WILL MAKE A HUGE DIFFERENCE.

A DIY MANICURE
*Give your hands a treat and
follow these easy steps for a
professional-looking manicure.*

1 Start by exfoliating your hands to
get rid of any hard, dry skin. You
can use a hand scrub, but a regular
body scrub will do the job just as well.
Rub it between your palms and between
your fingers too so that you don't miss
any areas.

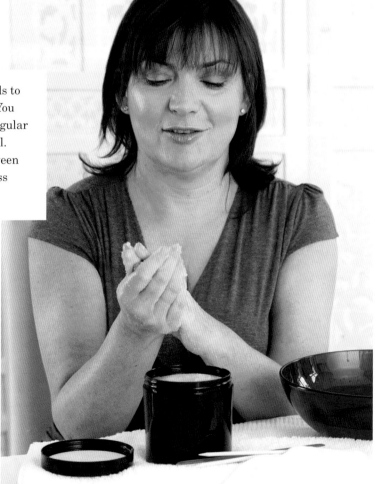

2 Wash your hands in warm water to remove the scrub and dry them carefully.

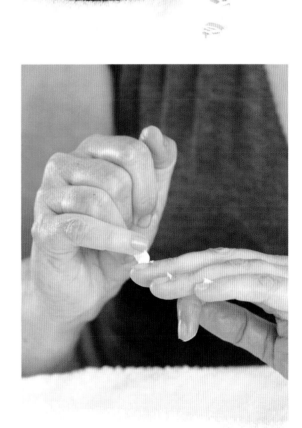

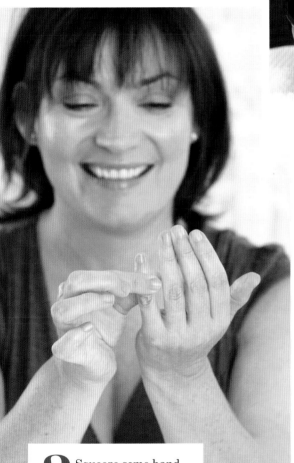

3 Squeeze some hand cream on to your hands. Moving from knuckle to tip, massage the cream into each finger in little circles. Really work it into the cuticle area and between the fingers.

4 Dab a tiny bit of cuticle cream on to each nail in turn and take the time massage it well into the cuticle.

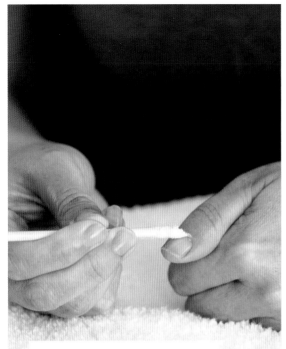

GOOD HAND HABITS

- Once a week give your hands a treat. Exfoliate, slather on the moisturizer and wear a pair of cotton gloves to bed. The next day your hands will be beautifully smooth.

- Keep a tub of body scrub beside the kitchen sink and exfoliate your hands whenever you feel they need a boost.

- Apply a sun block to the backs of your hands each day, to protect them from sun damage.

- To keep nails healthy, make sure you include plenty of iron, zinc and vitamins A and D in your diet (see pages 12–13).

- Protect your hands by wearing warm gloves in winter and always wear rubber gloves to do the washing up.

- Keep tubes of hand cream in the car, in your bag, on the bedside table and in your desk drawer at work so that you're reminded to moisturize your hands often.

5 Wrap a small piece of cotton wool around the flat end of an orange stick and moisten the cotton wool with cuticle remover. Use soft, circular motions to lift any dry, dead skin off the nails. Be gentle and take care not to scratch the nail bed.

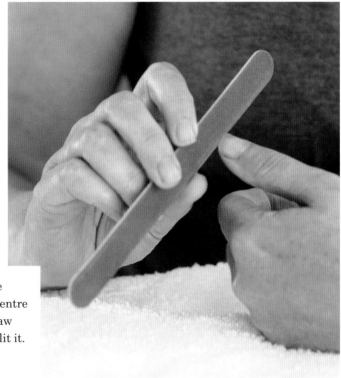

6 File each nail from the outside corner to the centre on either side. Don't saw across the nail as this can split it.

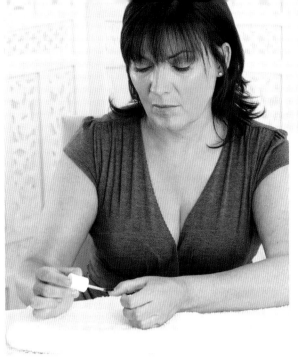

7 Apply a base-coat polish. A base coat stops coloured polish from staining the nails and also helps to hold the coloured polish for longer. Use three vertical strokes to cover the nail and finish with a horizontal stroke of base coat across the top of the nail. The combination of horizontal and vertical strokes will also help your nail polish to last for longer and stop it from peeling off too easily.

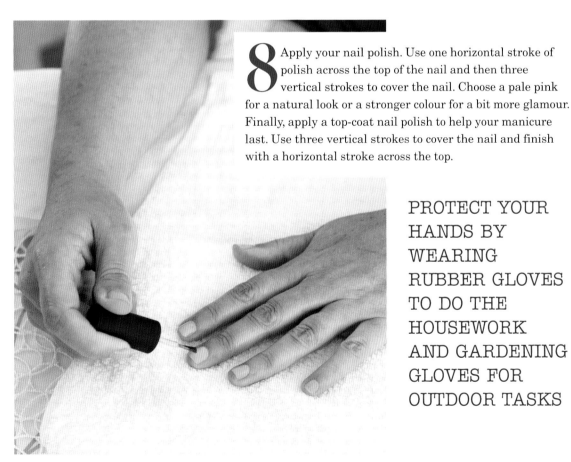

8 Apply your nail polish. Use one horizontal stroke of polish across the top of the nail and then three vertical strokes to cover the nail. Choose a pale pink for a natural look or a stronger colour for a bit more glamour. Finally, apply a top-coat nail polish to help your manicure last. Use three vertical strokes to cover the nail and finish with a horizontal stroke across the top.

PROTECT YOUR HANDS BY WEARING RUBBER GLOVES TO DO THE HOUSEWORK AND GARDENING GLOVES FOR OUTDOOR TASKS

Fabulous feet

MY FEET ARE NOT EXACTLY MY BEST
FEATURE, ESPECIALLY SINCE I STARTED DOING
MARATHONS AND LONG-DISTANCE CHARITY
WALKS. SINCE THEN I HAVE TRIED TO GIVE
MYSELF A HOME PEDICURE ONCE A WEEK,
ESPECIALLY IN THE SUMMER WHEN YOU WANT
TO BE WEARING OPEN-TOE SHOES.

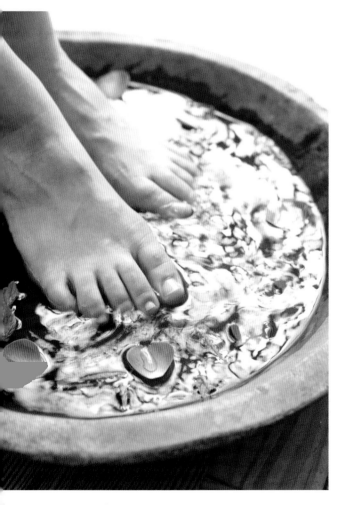

HEALTHY FEET

We tend to neglect our feet a bit, especially in winter when they're hidden inside boots and comfy socks, but they deserve better. Paying regular attention to your feet is more effective than a sudden attack on cracked heels or corns when summer arrives.

Remove rough, hard skin regularly to make your feet feel softer and to reinvigorate healthy cell growth. Pumice stones and foot files are great for this. Use an even, regular rubbing motion and don't push down too hard or put pressure in the same place for too long. Follow this up with an exfoliating foot scrub for extra-soft feet, and don't forget to moisturize feet and ankles daily.

Keep toenails in shape by trimming them regularly. Use nail clippers and always trim straight across, following the natural shape of the nail. Don't try to cut around the corners of nails as this might encourage ingrowing toenails. Don't cut too close to the skin, as this can cause soreness and possibly infection. It's easier to clip toenails when they're damp, so do this after showering or a warm bath.

Feet need exercise to stay healthy – this will strengthen muscles, lift arches and improve circulation – and one of the very best things you can do for your feet is walking.

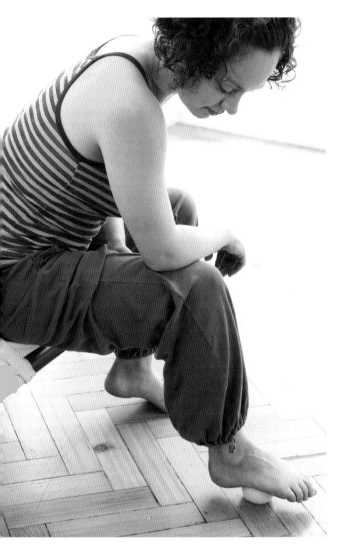

TREAT YOUR FEET

After a long day, revitalize hot, tired feet with one of these pick-me-ups:

Foot and leg massage Lie down with your feet propped up on a pillow about 20 cm (8 in) above your head for 15 minutes. Then, using sweet almond massage oil or invigorating peppermint foot cream, gently massage each leg from foot to knee, working upwards.

Foot bath Add a tablespoon of chopped fresh mint or rosemary to about 2.5 litres (4 pints) of boiling water in a large basin or bucket. Leave to cool down for 15 minutes and then sit comfortably with both feet immersed in the water and just relax for a while.

Ball rolling Rolling a tennis ball under each foot for a few minutes is a surprisingly effective way of soothing sore feet (sit down to do this to avoid accidents!).

GREAT-LOOKING FEET

Here are my tips for making the most of your feet:

- I love high heels and sparkly, crazy shoes, but you need to make sure they fit you properly or you will get blisters, bunions and corns.
- Slather cream on your feet, pop on some socks and sleep in them. In the morning your feet will be as smooth as a baby's bottom.
- If you are wearing your favourite pair of high heels, add one of those cushions to the instep and you will be able to dance the night away.

- Painting your toenails gives you a real boost and the nail polish lasts at least twice as long as it does on your fingernails. You can also get away with really sassy colours on your feet.
- Give yourself an instant pedicure on holiday by walking barefoot in the sand – make sure you put plenty of sun block on your feet first.
- When applying cream make sure that you cover the top of your feet and around the ankle area, too, as well as the bottoms of your feet.

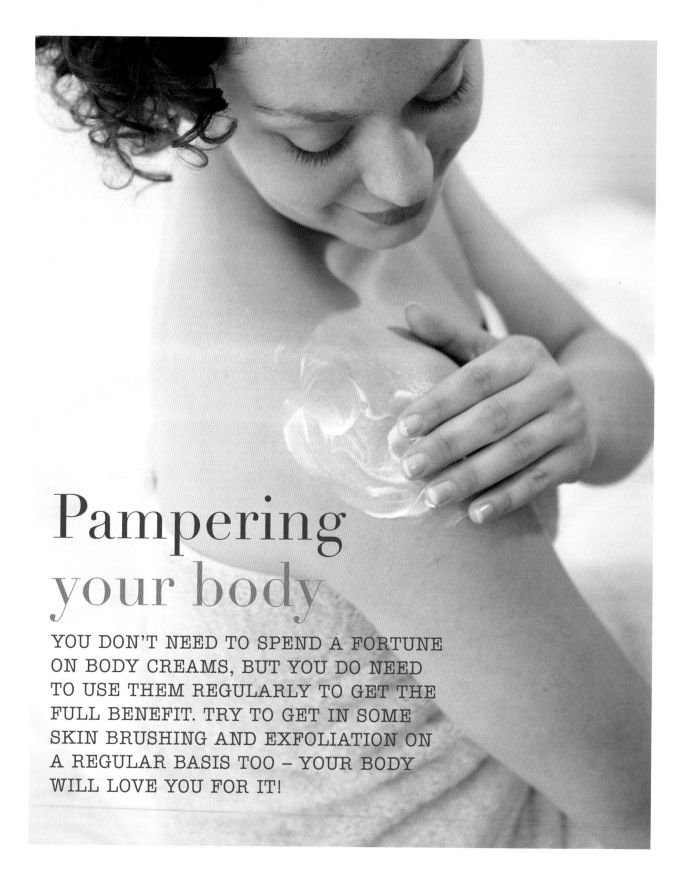

Pampering
your body

YOU DON'T NEED TO SPEND A FORTUNE
ON BODY CREAMS, BUT YOU DO NEED
TO USE THEM REGULARLY TO GET THE
FULL BENEFIT. TRY TO GET IN SOME
SKIN BRUSHING AND EXFOLIATION ON
A REGULAR BASIS TOO – YOUR BODY
WILL LOVE YOU FOR IT!

MOISTURIZING

To keep your skin soft and hydrated, make moisturizing your whole body part of your daily routine. I find the best time to do this is straight after my morning shower when my skin is freshly clean. To help your skin absorb body lotion better, don't dry yourself off completely. Just pat yourself dry and then gently massage in the body lotion, paying particular attention to areas where skin is very dry – often elbows and ankles – and where the skin is thinner, like your chest.

In winter, when skin tends to be more thirsty, you might want to go for a richer body moisturizer, perhaps with shea butter or cocoa butter. In summer, you could choose a lighter body lotion that incorporates an SPF.

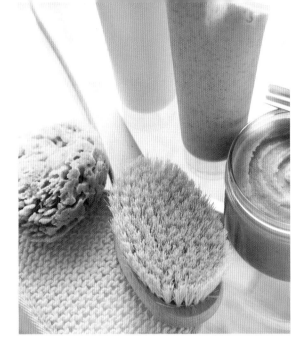

EXFOLIATING

Exfoliating regularly is terrific for overall skin health – it sloughs away dead skin cells so that your skin is smoother and fresher, and boosts circulation too. It's also vital to exfoliate before you apply fake tan to avoid that unattractive stripy look. You can use an exfoliating scrub or an exfoliating sponge/body cloth with your favourite shower gel.

SKIN BRUSHING

Skin brushing is a great way to make your skin smooth and glowing, as it removes the top layer of dull, dead skin. It also stimulates blood flow, which is really invigorating and helps to combat cellulite and eliminate toxins from your body. It's done on dry skin and you need to be firm enough to give yourself a bit of a tingle, but not so rough that you damage your skin.

FIVE-MINUTE SKIN BRUSHING

Why not invest in a long-handled body brush and follow this simple routine each morning?

1 Begin with the right foot. Use firm, rhythmic strokes to cover the top of your foot several times, brushing up towards your ankle. Then go on to your lower leg, making sure you cover both shin and calf, always brushing in an upward direction. Now brush from knee to thigh several times, using long strokes, and brush your buttock area as far as your waist. Now repeat on your left leg, starting at your left foot.

2 Then, starting from the buttocks and always moving upwards, brush the whole of your back several times all the way up to your shoulders.

3 Move on to brush the palm of your right hand. Move to the back of the hand and, always moving upwards, brush from your wrist to your elbow and from your elbow, along your upper arm, to your shoulder. Make sure you cover the whole surface of your arm several times. Repeat on your left side.

4 Very gently, brush your abdomen several times in a clockwise direction. Use less pressure than you did on your arms and legs and stop if it feels uncomfortable.

5 The neck and chest are very sensitive, so brush these areas very carefully in a rhythmic motion, always working towards your heart.

Hair-care essentials

WHENEVER WE DO A MAKE-OVER FEATURE ON MY SHOW, IT'S ALWAYS THE NEW HAIRSTYLE THAT REALLY MAKES THE DIFFERENCE TO THE 'AFTER' LOOK. SO MANY WOMEN STICK TO A STYLE THAT THEY HAVE SIMPLY GROWN OUT OF AND WHICH DOESN'T DO THEM JUSTICE.

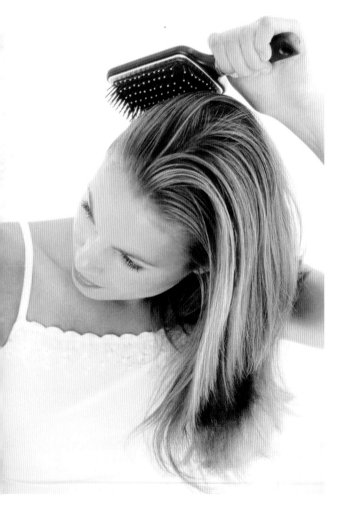

CUT

An expert haircut is easily the best beauty present you can give yourself. A clever cut can emphasize your best features and disguise your bad ones, so don't be afraid – talk to your stylist about a style that will update your look and enhance your face and go for it!

Many women in their 30s, 40s and older have stuck to the same style for decades but you need to adapt your look as you get older. A new haircut, and perhaps some great colour, will take years off you and give you a real confidence boost.

COLOUR

Deciding whether to colour your hair is a personal thing. Some women look stunning with grey or white hair cut in a chic style. But, if you're not ready to go grey just yet, choosing to zap it away and lift your look is something I would recommend to any woman.

The trick when you're deciding what colour to go for is to find something that complements your natural skin tone and your eye colour. This can be difficult to get absolutely right so, unless your budget is very tight or you are confident in selecting the best colour, it is well worth seeing a professional colourist who will help you choose a flattering shade.

IF YOUR HAIR LOOKS GOOD, YOU'LL LOOK GOOD, NO MATTER WHAT YOU'RE WEARING OR HOW LITTLE MAKE-UP YOU HAVE ON

FABULOUS HAIR

Here are my tips for making the most of your hair:

- Having a good cut or a dramatic recolouring can take years off you and it is well worth the investment of going to a good stylist for proper advice and a real professional job.

- If you do home hair colour, always make sure that you do a test for any allergic reaction first.

- Be kind to wet hair. Towel-dry it gently and take time to detangle knots. Use a wide-toothed comb, rather than a brush, on wet hair to avoid stretching it.

- Brush your hair before washing it to massage the scalp and help to loosen dead skin cells.

- Avoid washing your hair more than once a day. More often than that, and you'll be stripping away the natural oils that help to make your hair thick and glossy.

- Keep your hairdryer on the lowest possible setting to minimize the damage the heat will do to your hair.

- Don't keep the hairdryer on one spot for too long. Keep it moving and hold it at a good distance away from your hair.

- Finish blow-drying your hair with a blast of cold air. This closes the cuticles, and when cuticles lie flat the hair reflects the light and makes it look shinier.

- Use hairspray to hold styled hair in place. To get a soft finish, rather than that rigid, 'crash helmet' effect that looks so ageing, spray into the palm of your hand and then smooth over the surface of the hair to control flyaway strands.

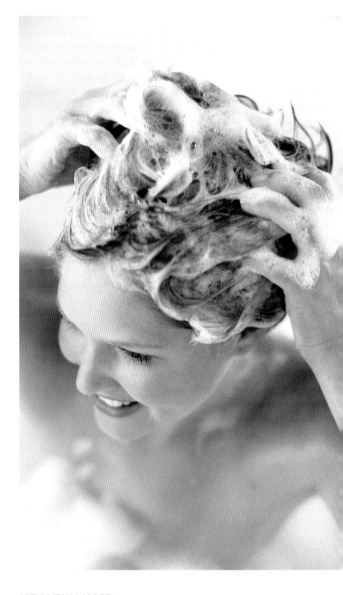

HEALTHY HAIR

Strong, shiny hair is down to much more than choosing the right shampoo and conditioner. Like the rest of your body, your scalp and hair need a balanced, nutritious diet with vitamins, minerals and other nutrients. You need to include plenty of essential fatty acids – found in things like nuts and seeds – to aid the production of sebum, which is what naturally lubricates your hair. Drinking plenty of water each day is also essential for glossy tresses.

Make-up know-how

I HAVE TO WEAR AN AWFUL LOT OF MAKE-UP WHEN I APPEAR ON GMTV, BUT I PUT ON MUCH LESS IN REAL LIFE. OF COURSE THE MOST DIFFICULT MAKE-UP JOB TO ACHIEVE IS THAT GLOWING, FRESH-FACED, 'NATURAL' LOOK.

m y mum and my aunt Josephine divide their make-up looks into a 'small' face, which is when you are just nipping out to the shops and slap on a bit of powder and lip gloss, and a 'big' face – the full works, even false eyelashes.

A NATURAL DAY-TIME LOOK

A 'natural' look appears effortless, but it can take twice as long as doing your make-up when you are going out on a special occasion. Here's how to achieve a fresh-faced appearance.

TOOLS OF THE TRADE

To get a flawless, professional finish to your make-up, you need to use the right brushes. Natural bristle brushes are gentler on the skin than synthetic ones. Buy the very best that you can afford, look after them and they'll last for years. The basic brushes you'll need are:

- Foundation brush
- Concealer brush
- Powder brush
- Eye shadow brushes – a small, angled one and a larger one
- Lip brush

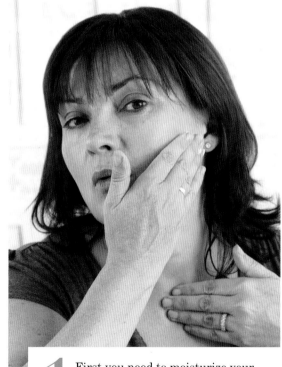

1 First you need to moisturize your face. Squeeze some moisturizer on to your hands and rub it between your fingers. Massage the moisturizer on to your skin, starting at your upper chest and working upwards (up your neck, across your cheeks and up to your brow, avoiding the eye area).

2 Next, you need to use primer. This helps your make-up last all day. Squeeze some primer on to your hand and rub it between your fingers. Massage the primer on to your skin, starting at your throat and working upwards in the same way as you did for the moisturizer.

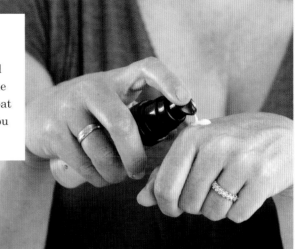

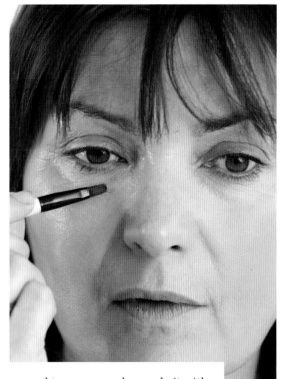

3 Squeeze some foundation on to your hand and rub it between your fingers. Press the foundation on to your face and gently massage it into your skin, working it into any creases. You can also use a wedge or brush to apply foundation. You may need to apply a little to your throat, particularly underneath your chin. People often have paler skin here, where it doesn't catch the sun.

4 If you need to use concealer, apply it with a brush. Using the flat part of the brush, gently apply the concealer with a patting motion, working in a 'C' shape from the corner of your eye and under your eye on both sides.

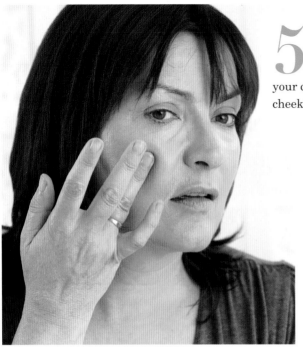

5 Dab some cream blusher on to the tip of your ring finger. Then gently pat it on to your skin, starting from the apples of your cheeks and working upwards along the cheekbones.

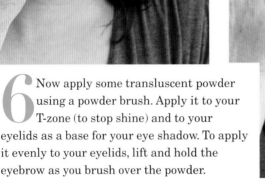

6 Now apply some transluscent powder using a powder brush. Apply it to your T-zone (to stop shine) and to your eyelids as a base for your eye shadow. To apply it evenly to your eyelids, lift and hold the eyebrow as you brush over the powder.

MY MAKE-UP TIPS

- Your foundation should match your skin tone. When choosing a foundation, always test it on your face rather than your wrist and go outside to see how it looks in daylight.

- Don't apply mascara to your bottom lashes. Alternatively, use brown on the bottom lashes and black on the top lashes.

- Most cosmetics counters keep samples of their products. Don't be afraid to ask for one so that you can try before you buy.

- Clean out your make-up bag regularly and throw away anything that has been lurking in there for ages.

- Make sure you clean your make-up brushes regularly.

- Keep your eyebrows in good shape: well-groomed eyebrows can give you an instant face lift.

- Try a new shade of eye shadow today. We all tend to stick with shades we used in our younger days but it is fun to experiment.

- A white kohl eyeliner on the inner eyelid can make your eyes 'pop' and look bigger and brighter, especially if they are a bit tired.

- Don't overdo the concealer, especially under your eyes, as this can actually draw attention to dark circles and eye bags.

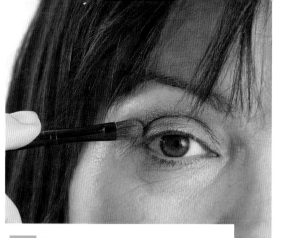

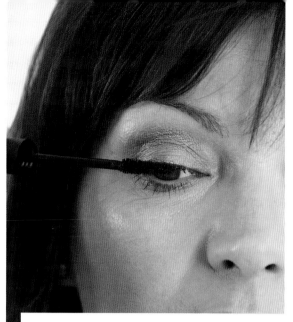

7 Using a large eye shadow brush, apply a light brown colour to your eye lid. Start at the inner corner and work out and up, applying all over the eye and socket area. Using a smaller eye shadow brush, apply a slightly darker brown colour just above the socket line. Start at the edge of the eye and take it up over the socket line. For a very natural look, take a bit of this darker colour under the eye.

8 Now you need to add mascara. Start with the bottom lashes and, once they're dry, apply mascara to the top lashes. You should start from the root of the lashes and move out towards the tips of the lashes in a zigzag movement.

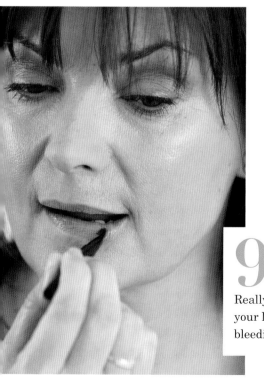

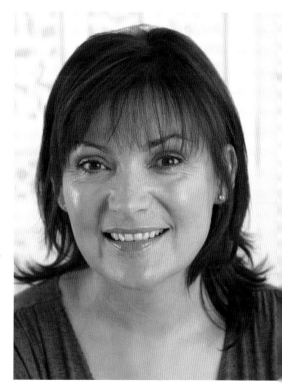

9 Finally, use a lip brush to apply a coloured lip gloss to your lips. Really work the gloss into your lips to avoid the colour bleeding.

Evening make-up

THIS IS WHEN YOU CAN HAVE FUN AND DO A
'BIG' FACE, BUT DON'T OVERDO IT. I LOVE
MAKING BIG, DRAMATIC EYES AND I ALWAYS
PUT MY EYE MAKE-UP ON BEFORE APPLYING
FOUNDATION SO THAT I CAN WIPE AWAY ANY
EYE SHADOW THAT SPILLS UNDER MY EYES.

I always use a primer before my foundation when I am going out at night. It gives a flawless base and my make-up lasts so much longer. Always remember to blend your foundation to avoid looking as if you are wearing a mask and, if you have a low-cut dress on, make sure you give your boobs a bit of colour and powder, too, so that everything matches.

A GLAMOROUS EVENING LOOK
Follow this step-by-step sequence to turn your natural day-time look (see pages 140–143) into a deeper, more sophisticated look for evenings out.

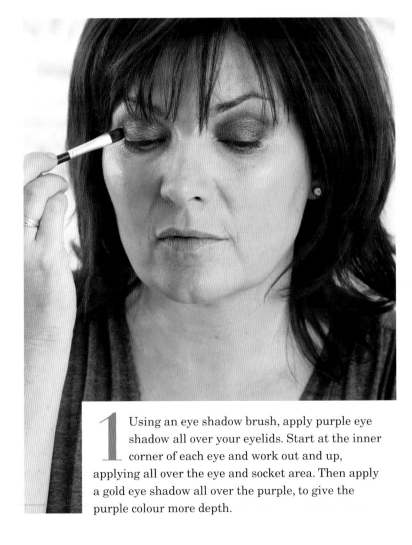

1 Using an eye shadow brush, apply purple eye shadow all over your eyelids. Start at the inner corner of each eye and work out and up, applying all over the eye and socket area. Then apply a gold eye shadow all over the purple, to give the purple colour more depth.

2 Blend a stronger smoky colour, such as a grey, into the corner of your eyelid. Use this stronger colour as eyeliner on the top lid and take it under the eye as well.

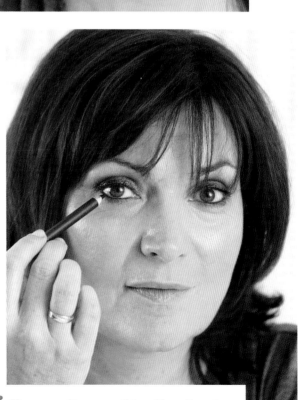

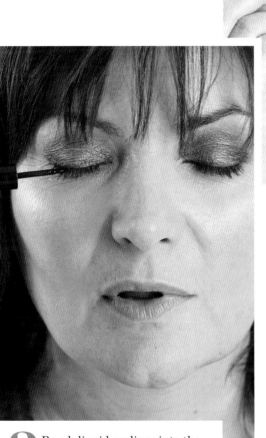

3 Brush liquid eyeliner into the base of your lashes by resting the brush on the lashes and just touching the skin. This enhances the thickness of your lashes but won't leave a defined, harsh line.

4 Use an eyeliner pencil to add eyeliner to the bottom of your eye. You might want to use a glitter eyeliner for a party look.

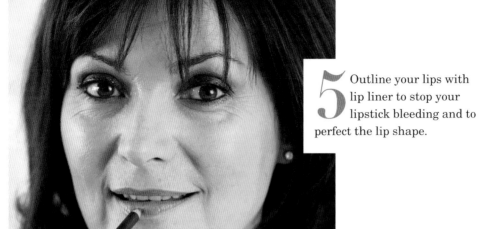

5 Outline your lips with lip liner to stop your lipstick bleeding and to perfect the lip shape.

6 Using a lip brush, apply a lipstick that is just a bit darker than your natural lip colour.

I DON'T LIKE
BRIGHT RED
LIPSTICK, AS I
FIND IT LOOKS
VERY AGEING
ON ME

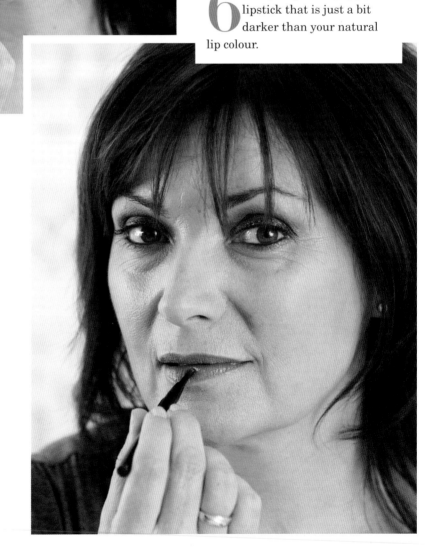

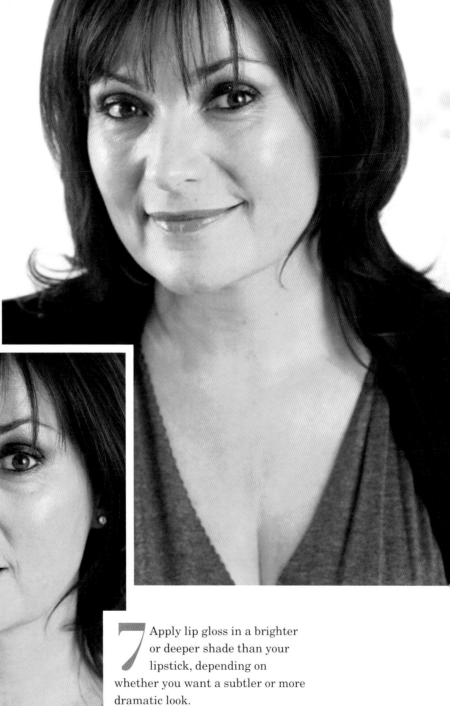

I REALLY LIKE
A BIT OF DARK
GLOSS ON TOP
OF A GOOD,
STRONG
LIPSTICK

7 Apply lip gloss in a brighter
or deeper shade than your
lipstick, depending on
whether you want a subtler or more
dramatic look.

Anti-ageing make-up

IT'S A FACT THAT AS WE GET OLDER OUR
SKIN CHANGES COLOUR AND TEXTURE AND
THE FEATURES ON OUR FACES CHANGE TOO –
FOR INSTANCE, LIPS BECOME LESS FULL – SO
PRODUCTS THAT LOOKED GREAT ON YOU TEN
YEARS AGO WON'T NECESSARILY MAKE YOU
LOOK YOUR BEST NOW.

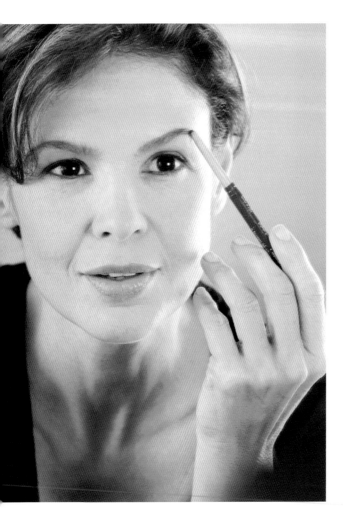

the good news is that there are some fantastic light-reflecting concealers and foundations around. With these, and other products made especially for more mature skin, you can really achieve a gorgeous look, no matter what age you are. It is well worth experimenting.

There's one rule when it comes to anti-ageing make-up: less is more. Trust me, the less make-up you apply, and the more natural it looks, the younger you will appear.

YOUR SKIN

As you get older it can be tempting to try to hide uneven skin tone and wrinkles under a heavier layer of foundation but this is a big mistake – instead of disguising wrinkles, a heavy mask of foundation will accentuate them. It is much better to apply a sheer foundation very lightly on your face and blend it well, keeping it from any crow's feet around your eyes (it tends to settle here, drawing attention to the lines). As skin often becomes drier with age, go for a moisturizing foundation that will keep your skin hydrated.

Primer is your secret weapon: it reflects light, which makes you look younger, evens out skin tone, fills in rough patches and wrinkles and makes foundation glide on smoothly. Use powder sparingly just along the T-zone to mop up any

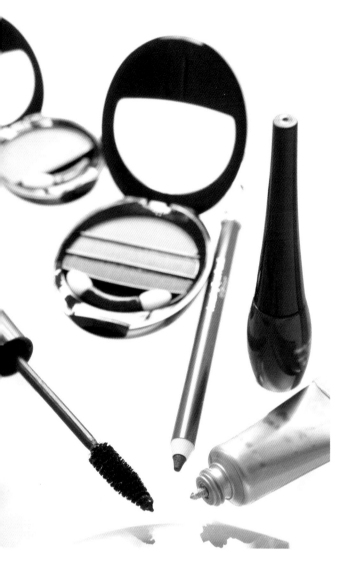

MAGIC TRICKS

It's amazing what make-up can do. Try my tips for looking your best as you get older:

- Always apply make-up in natural daylight or using strong artificial light that doesn't cast any shadows on your face, so that you can really see what you're doing and how it looks.

- I use creamy eye shadows, which tend to crease less around the eyes.

- I prefer to use a cream blusher, rather than powder blusher, as it is hydrating and gives a more youthful, dewy look.

- Use a light, translucent face powder that won't clog up your pores and emphasize any wrinkles.

- Fake tan is so much less ageing than sitting in the sun, and a good tinted moisturizer looks good on holiday. You will find it lighter than wearing moisturizer and foundation. Check it has a high enough SPF to protect your skin.

If you have fine wrinkles around your mouth, use a lip liner in a nude shade to outline your lips before you put on lipstick to stop the lipstick bleeding into the wrinkles.

YOUR EYES

Black eyeliner and mascara look harsh and heavy on a mature face – change to a more flattering shade of brown or grey, instead.

Eyelashes and eyebrows both tend to become more sparse and faded with age, so choose a volumizing mascara to give lashes lots of body, and apply it only to your upper lashes for a more natural look. Carefully fill in sparse brows with a brow pencil or brow shadow in a shade that matches your natural eyebrow colour. If your brows become very pale, consider dyeing them.

I would suggest that you opt for a neutral palette, such as taupe, soft greys and browns for eye shadow, to get a natural, flattering effect and avoid shimmery and frosted eye shadow which will highlight crêpe-like eyelids.

shine. Too much powder on the face gathers in lines and wrinkles and makes them more noticeable.

YOUR LIPS

Lips lose their colour and get thinner as we get older and our bodies produce less collagen. Give your lips a boost by applying a creamy, hydrating lipstick – avoid matt and frosted lipsticks, which will age you – and finish by adding a touch of gloss to the middle of your bottom lip. This will reflect light and create the effect of fullness.

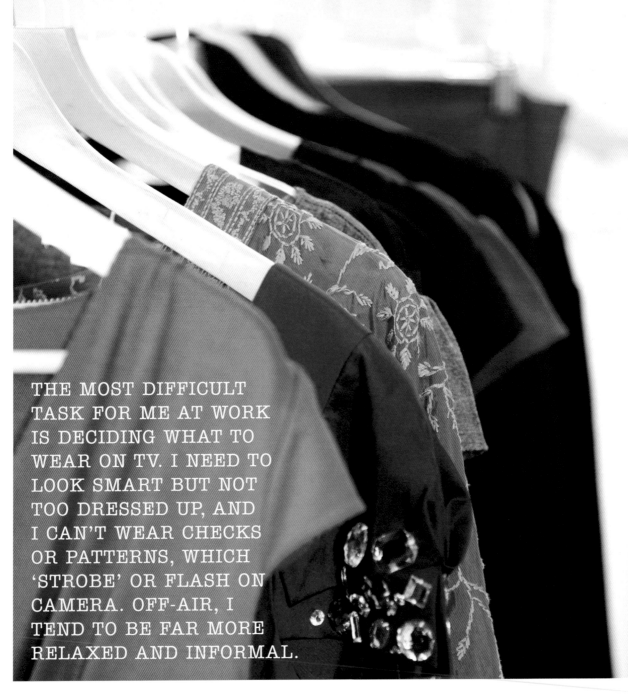

Wardrobe essentials

THE MOST DIFFICULT TASK FOR ME AT WORK IS DECIDING WHAT TO WEAR ON TV. I NEED TO LOOK SMART BUT NOT TOO DRESSED UP, AND I CAN'T WEAR CHECKS OR PATTERNS, WHICH 'STROBE' OR FLASH ON CAMERA. OFF-AIR, I TEND TO BE FAR MORE RELAXED AND INFORMAL.

It took me until my 40s to find a look I am happy with and I have made some howlers in my time. Take my advice and use the following basic steps in building a collection of clothes that will see you through any event, day or night.

WHAT EVERY WOMAN SHOULD OWN

We all have days when we stand in front of the wardrobe wailing that we 'don't have a thing to wear'. You can have fewer of those days by making sure you own some of these key items:

Black trousers A pair of well-cut black trousers in a fabric that will last and drape well, such as fine wool, is a wise investment.

Cashmere cardigan A soft cashmere cardie adds a bit of luxury and, looked after properly, lasts for ages.

Killer heels Even if you're normally the tracksuit and trainers type, you need one pair of absolutely gorgeous heels.

Little black dress Floaty and feminine or sexy and satin, every woman simply has to have the perfect little black dress.

Jeans Shop around until you find the perfect pair for you. The right jeans will make your legs look longer and your bottom look smaller, whatever size or shape you are.

Tailored jacket Choose one that's cut properly so that it sits neatly across your shoulders and buttons comfortably. Go for a multi-use, neutral colour, such as black, grey or camel.

Trench coat A classic trench coat never goes out of fashion and will make you feel and look sophisticated.

White shirt Crisp and classy, a white shirt goes with everything from jeans to an interview outfit and can be worn whatever the season.

White T-shirt These tend to get dingy-looking quickly and need to be snowy white to look good so don't waste money on expensive designer ones; it's better to buy cheaper ones more often.

> I LIKE TO WEAR A LOT OF CASUAL CLOTHES IN SOFT, COMFORTABLE FABRICS

SPECIAL OCCASIONS

Getting all dressed up for a special occasion is tremendous fun, but many women worry about getting it right. Here are a few pointers for stylish ways to put on the glitz.

To get the most for your money, aim to buy something versatile and timeless, which you'll be able to accessorize in different ways and wear time and again. That doesn't mean you can't be comfortable. So, for example, if you prefer wearing trousers, by all means, do. Just make sure they're absolutely stunning and team them with a blouse or jacket in a luxurious fabric and great jewellery. However, grooming is vital – there's no point in wearing shoes to die for if you need a pedicure.

Resist the temptation to overmatch your accessories. Shoes that exactly match your bag will make your outfit look dated and less individual.

WARDROBE WORK-OUT

Here's some advice on how to keep your wardrobe under control:

- Make sure you have the basics and build outfits around them.
- You don't need to spend a fortune on clothes, but it is worth investing in a little black dress that will still be fashionable when you are in your 80s.
- Never buy a designer outfit in a sale if it isn't your size or a colour you love.
- Do regular clear-outs and give the clothes to charity shops. If you haven't worn something for a year then, chances are, you never will.
- Don't be a slave to fashion and don't be afraid to try something a little bit different.
- If you are feeling a bit fed up, especially if you are having a 'plump' day, remember that your feet don't get fat and a new pair of shoes is always a real pick-me-up.

Accessories

ACCESSORIES CAN CHANGE AN OUTFIT FROM SO-SO TO SENSATIONAL. THEY NEEDN'T BE EXPENSIVE; IN FACT BUYING A NEW BELT OR BAG, RATHER THAN A NEW DRESS, IS OFTEN THE MOST AFFORDABLE WAY OF ENJOYING A LITTLE RETAIL THERAPY AND ADDING INDIVIDUALITY TO YOUR LOOK.

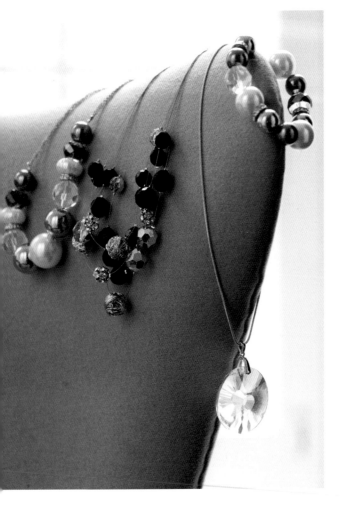

JEWELLERY

This is the quickest, and often cheapest, way to introduce this season's look and colours to your wardrobe. A funky necklace or fun bracelet is also a great way of making you look more youthful and adding a touch of trendy without overdoing it.

SCARVES

Scarves have a multitude of uses: a fast-fix cover-up for bad hair days, a splash of cheering colour with a dark winter coat and a stylish way to belt your jeans, for instance. It's worth investing in a selection of scarves in different colours, sizes and fabrics.

SHOES

All women love shoes and quite rightly so! A fabulous pair of shoes can transform an outfit and make you feel confident and sexy. Here are few things to bear in mind:

- Heels add length to your legs and make you look taller and slimmer. If really high heels just aren't for you, try kitten heels.
- Ankle straps only work if you have slim ankles. They can make your legs look shorter because, visually, they cut them in half.
- Boots – ankle, calf or knee-length – all need to finish at a slim point on your leg, otherwise

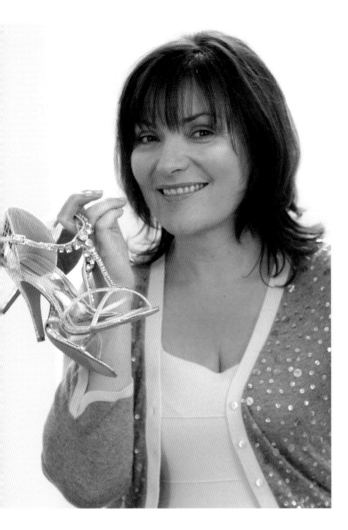

We all love a new bag or pair of heels, but keep the following tips in mind:

- Less can sometimes be more. Take care not to look like a Christmas tree by wearing too much bling.
- I love big bags, but do tend to over fill them and risk back injury. Be ruthless about what you carry around in your oversized bags.
- Check out the high-street shops for shoes. Many of them pay 'homage' to Jimmy Choo, Christian Louboutin and Gina at a fraction of the price.
- I do, however, think it is worth investing in at least one really good pair of high heels that fit properly and won't cause you pain and suffering.

can go with everything. Both have their place in your wardrobe. Different occasions call for different styles of handbag; try to build up a collection so that, whatever the occasion, you have the right bag.

BELTS

Belts can add detail and interest to whatever you're wearing and a well-chosen one can really bring an outfit together. For the most flattering look, there are a few things to think about:

- Narrow belts look best on slim waists.
- If you have a big tummy, wearing a belt around your hips will draw attention away from it.
- Dark belts in a matt material are the most slimming.
- For larger women, it's a good tip to opt for a belt in a similar colour to your clothing and avoid a strongly contrasting colour.

SUNGLASSES

These are essential for adding instant glamour to your look. Get a pair that flatter your face and make sure that they offer enough protection for your eyes.

they'll have the effect of making your legs look wider than they actually are.

- Comfy shoes don't have to be dowdy and old-ladyish – ballet pumps and flat boots, for example, can be both stylish and practical.
- Matching your shoe colour and the colour of your tights will help your legs look thinner and longer. If your skirt is also the same colour, the monochromatic effect will make you look thinner from the waist down.

BAGS

Bags can be a fun. An up-to-the minute version that costs under £20, or an investment piece in quality leather and a classic design that will last forever,

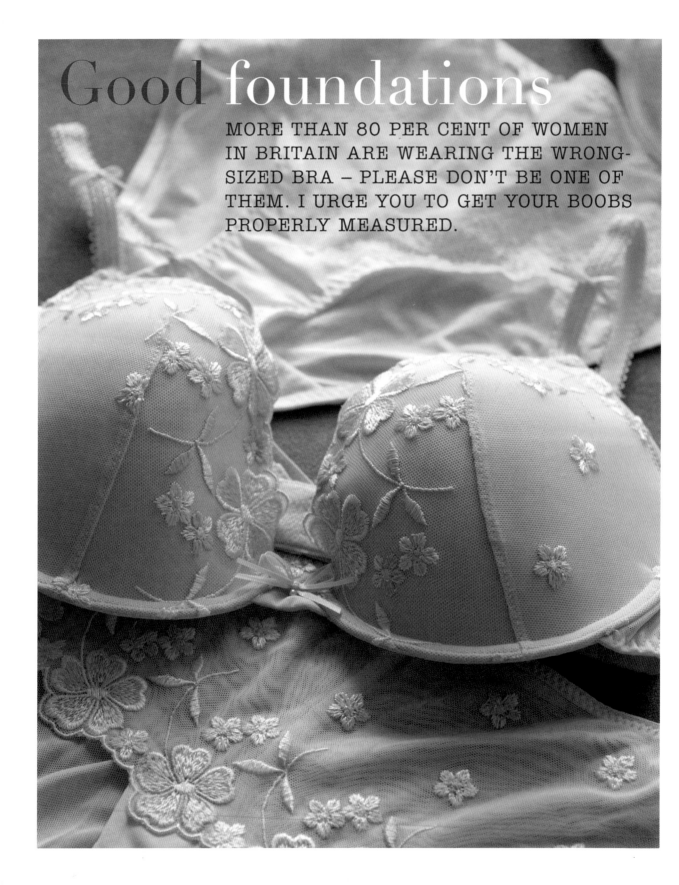

Good foundations

MORE THAN 80 PER CENT OF WOMEN IN BRITAIN ARE WEARING THE WRONG-SIZED BRA – PLEASE DON'T BE ONE OF THEM. I URGE YOU TO GET YOUR BOOBS PROPERLY MEASURED.

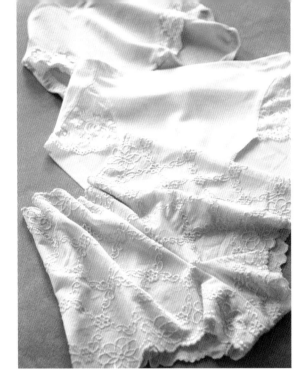

Proper underwear can take pounds off you and its worth investing in a good pair of Bridget Jones big knickers. They might not be sexy but they do the job beautifully and give you a confidence boost. Underwear can make or break an outfit, so spend some time and money on finding underwear that fits properly, provides the right coverage and support and doesn't reveal ugly bulges or seams.

YOUR BRA

Bodies change – they become bigger, smaller, older, droopier or fitter – and all of this means that your bra size can change, too. Most department stores and big chains offer a free bra measuring and fitting service so get yourself along there and find out what size you really are. You need to have patience to shop for a bra, in order to make sure that you get one that's right. Even if you know what size you are, there are differences between brands and styles, as is the case with most clothing, so here are a few tips:

- A bra that fits correctly should never pull, dig in or cause any discomfort.
- It should fit snugly but not tightly – you should be able to fit two fingers under the band comfortably.
- The centre of the bra should lie flat against your breastbone.
- Your breasts should fit comfortably in the cups and there should be a smooth line where the cup ends and it meets your breast.
- Wrinkly, baggy cups or any extra fabric means the cup size is too big.
- The strap around your back should be firm and should stay at the same level all the way around without riding up.
- When you buy a new bra, make sure it fits comfortably on the loosest hook, as you may need to tighten it as the bra stretches with washing and wear.
- The best way to see what a bra is doing for you is to check what it looks like under a fitted T-shirt. You should have smooth lines and no bulges.

KNICKERS!

There are numerous styles around and you should wear whatever makes you comfortable and works with the outfit, but – whether you go for French knickers or bikini briefs – there's one golden rule: no visible panty line (VPL), ever!

The other thing to remember is that, unless you want people to notice your underwear more than what you're wearing over it, flesh-coloured knickers are the way to go when you are wearing white or cream, especially trousers.

BODY SHAPERS

The secret beneath many a designer gown, body shapers are what give the stars their enviably svelte red-carpet look. Shapers can control your thighs, lift your bottom, flatten your tummy and make you look slimmer instantly. Unlike the corsets and girdles your granny was condemned to, they're comfortable, don't cut off your circulation and let you breathe and eat comfortably. Body shapers are available in a vast range of styles from knickers that hold in your tummy to all-in-one versions that gives your whole body a slimmer, smoother silhouette.

Dress right
for your shape

MOST OF US AREN'T A PERFECT SIZE 10,
12, 14 OR 16. WHEN I AM BUYING CLOTHES
THE SIZE I NEED DEPENDS ON WHAT SHOP I
GO INTO, BUT USUALLY I AM A SIZE 12 ON
THE TOP AND, MORE OFTEN THAN NOT, I AM
A 14 ON THE BOTTOM.

When it comes to looking good, wearing clothes that suit your shape is key. If you know how to make the most of your figure, whatever it is, you can choose clothes that flatter your best features and disguise the less-than-perfect ones.

I am more of an apple shape than a pear, and I need to take that into account when I am buying clothes so that I opt for clothes that draw the eye away from my round middle!

WHAT'S YOUR SHAPE?

All women will fit into one of the following body shape categories. It has nothing to do with what you weigh or what size clothes you wear – it's about proportion.

Pear This is the most common shape by far. You're a pear if your shoulders are narrower than your hips and your upper half is noticeably smaller – sometimes a size or two – than your bottom half. If you put on weight, it will mostly be on your hips and thighs.

TAKE YOUR BODY SHAPE INTO ACCOUNT WHEN BUYING CLOTHES AND CHOOSE GARMENTS THAT WILL MAKE THE MOST OF YOUR GOOD POINTS

Apple Also called an 'oval', this is a rounded shape, where the upper body tends to be broader than the lower. You have fullness in the tummy area and, if you put on weight, that's where it will go.

Hourglass This is the figure many women dream of! You're curvy, well proportioned and have a clearly defined waist. Any weight you might put on will tend to be evenly distributed around your body.

Rectangle Women with a rectangular shape are straight up and down, without many defined curves. If you put on any weight it will be evenly distributed.

Knowing your body shape and dressing to make the most of your good points will give you a whole new look and a lot more confidence. I like to cover the tops of my arms and my tummy and have invested in a number of little shrugs. Peplum skirts and dresses cut on the bias also flatter my shape.

Opposite is a guide to what to wear and what not to wear so that you feel comfortable and confident and look great.

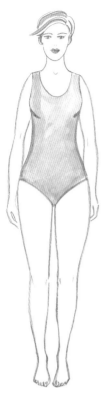
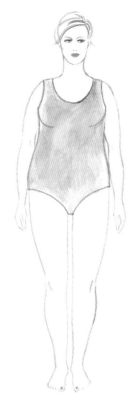
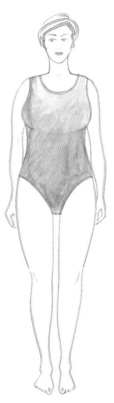
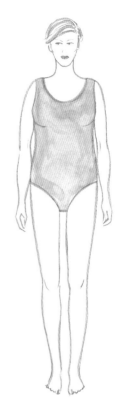

IF YOU'RE A PEAR

Do wear A-line skirts for a streamlined effect; eye-catching tops that draw attention upwards; bootleg and flared trousers to balance proportions; dark colours on your bottom half to minimize hips and thighs; wraparound dresses; three-quarter-length coats and jackets that skim over your hips.

Avoid Anything with side pockets; tops and jackets that stop at your widest point; shift dresses; super-slim jeans; pencil skirts.

IF YOU'RE AN APPLE

Do wear Tops and dresses that have interest at the neckline to draw attention from the stomach; flat-fronted trousers and side-fastening skirts to avoid adding bulk around the middle; soft fabrics; trousers with a simple silhouette; tops with scoop necks.

Avoid Clingy fabrics; gathered waistlines; tops tucked into trousers or skirts.

IF YOU'RE AN HOURGLASS

Do wear Pencil skirts; waist-length jackets and tops; belted coats and jackets; dresses that define your waist; belts.

Avoid Baggy sweaters and tops which will make you look lumpy not curvy; straight tunics; boxy jackets.

IF YOU'RE A RECTANGLE

Do wear Slim-fitting and straight-legged jeans and trousers; tops with gathers at sleeves or waist detailing to break up the straight lines; wide belts to give more definition at the waistline; wraparound dresses; tops with neck detailing to draw the eye up.

Avoid Pencil skirts; shift dresses; straight-lined and boxy jackets, all of which emphasize the straight lines of your shape.

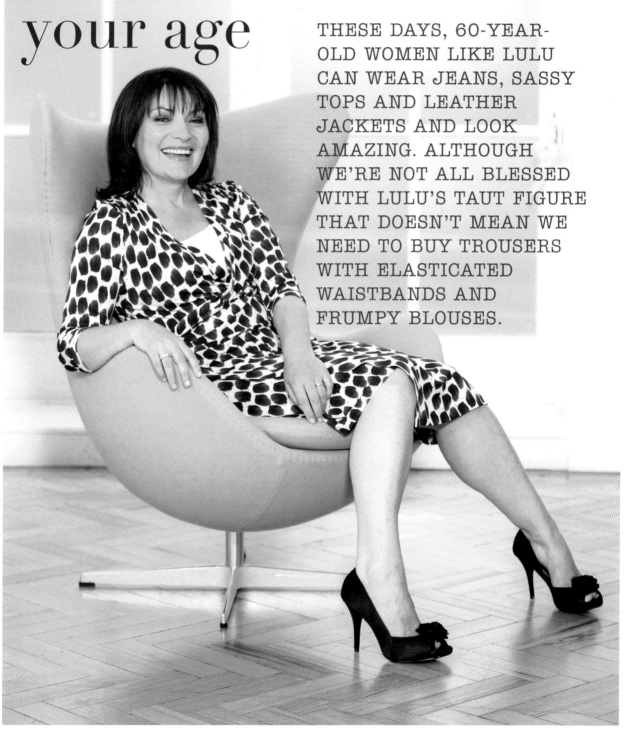

Dressing for your age

THESE DAYS, 60-YEAR-OLD WOMEN LIKE LULU CAN WEAR JEANS, SASSY TOPS AND LEATHER JACKETS AND LOOK AMAZING. ALTHOUGH WE'RE NOT ALL BLESSED WITH LULU'S TAUT FIGURE THAT DOESN'T MEAN WE NEED TO BUY TROUSERS WITH ELASTICATED WAISTBANDS AND FRUMPY BLOUSES.

I had to take the tough decision to get rid of my tartan mini kilt when I hit my late 40s because it was just too short and too young for me. I still wear a tartan skirt, but now it's a tight-fitting pencil skirt that comes just above the knee and I wear it with a crisp black or white blouse, black tights and high heels. It looks elegant, a bit cheeky, but does not give the impression that I am trying too hard.

There are no hard-and-fast rules about age-appropriate dressing: the key is to wear clothes that fit well, look good and make you feel confident. There are, however, some things you could bear in mind when you're out shopping for clothes.

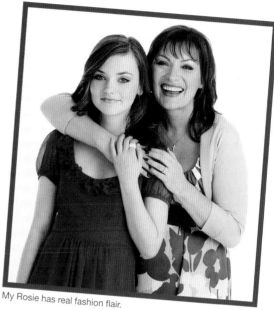
My Rosie has real fashion flair.

FASHION

You'll look younger for longer if you stay in touch with trends in fashion. You can do this by reading magazines, browsing in the shops and on the Internet, and simply by observing what people are wearing on your local high street. Be wary of sticking slavishly to fashionable trends, however; this is what teenagers do and will make you a fashion victim – be selective instead, and pick only those elements of current fashion that you know will look good on you.

COLOUR

There are two aspects of colour that you need to be aware of. The first is how to wear black. Black is a

useful wardrobe staple, but you need to wear it with care as you get older – it tends to look harsh and ageing worn near the face. It's more flattering to wear black below the waist and, if you do want to wear a black dress or top, break it up with a colourful scarf or necklace.

The second thing to remember is: don't be afraid of colour. Just because you're older, it doesn't mean you need to play it safe with matronly pastels. Adding a splash of a jewel colour – such as scarlet, emerald, acid yellow or rich purple – will give you an instant youthful edge and a dash of panache.

SHOWING SKIN

How much skin to show as you age is a matter of personal choice but, unless your body is in the most fantastic shape, miniskirts and bare midriffs are things to steer clear of. Many women in the UK worry about their flabby upper arms and, if you have this problem, sleeveless tops and dresses are best avoided, too.

Two parts of the body that tend not to age and so are good points to draw attention to are your wrists and your collarbones. Think about getting the focus on slim wrists with a bracelet or sleeve detail and highlight collarbones with a flattering slash-neck top.

LOOKING GREAT AT ANY AGE

Don't ever think that, because you are no longer a teenager, you need to be a fashion frump. You don't want to look like mutton dressed as lamb but you also don't want to be old before your time.

You can still shop in trendy shops – just be choosy and don't go for the whole 'look'.

Bags and shoes can jazz up an outfit and make you look trendy and sassy without appearing desperate to look young.

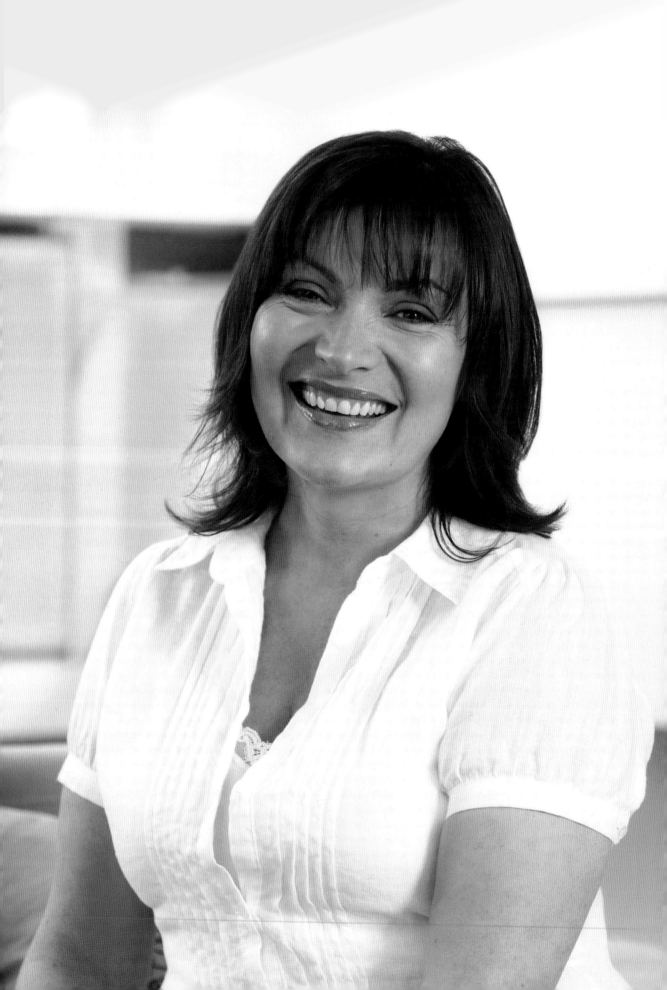

STAYING HEALTHY

Be breast aware

MY GRANDMOTHER DIED OF BREAST CANCER AND, ALTHOUGH SHE WAS IN HER 80S, I STILL FEEL CHEATED THAT SHE NEVER GOT TO SEE MY DAUGHTER. SHE LEFT IT TOO LATE TO ASK FOR HELP, WHICH IS WHY I DO WHAT I CAN TO PROMOTE SELF-EXAMINATION AND AWARENESS OF BREAST CANCER.

two very good friends of mine each discovered lumps in their breasts, went to their GPs immediately and received swift and excellent treatment. They both went through a rough time, but are now absolutely fit and fabulous, but only because they chose not to ignore their symptoms.

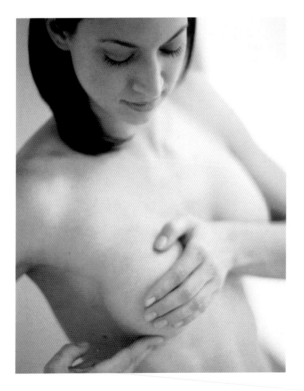

WHO GETS BREAST CANCER?

Breast cancer can affect any of us – men and women alike – but there are some things that can either raise or lower your risk. It's important to remember, though, that even if you fall into one or more of these categories, it doesn't mean that you will go on to develop cancer.

Age This is biggest risk factor; in the UK over 80 per cent of breast cancer cases are women over the age of 50.

Relatives Having a close member of the family (mother, daughter or sister) with breast cancer increases your risk.

Breastfeeding Women who have never breastfed are more at risk than those who choose to breastfeed their babies.

Menstruation An early first period and late menopause are both associated with higher risk.

Body weight Obesity and being overweight, particularly after the menopause, increases breast cancer risk.

Alcohol Excessive boozing pushes your risk up.

Hormone replacement therapy (HRT) This is thought to increase the risk very slightly.

Exercise A sedentary lifestyle can increase the risk of breast cancer. Studies have shown that being physically active can lower your risk by up to one-third.

IT IS BETTER TO BE SAFE
THAN SORRY; THE EARLIER
ANY PROBLEMS ARE
DETECTED THE GREATER
YOUR CHANCES OF A
COMPLETE CURE.

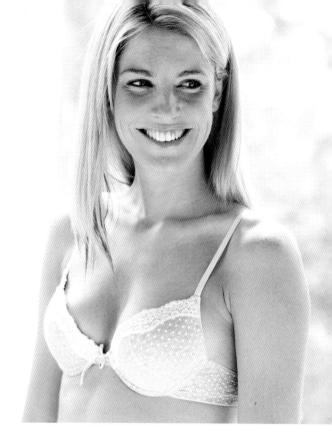

Diet A diet high in saturated fat can increase your risk, while opting for less saturated fat and a diet that has plenty of fibre, calcium and foods rich in carotenoids, including tomatoes, carrots, sweet potatoes and spinach, can lower your risk.

THE FIVE-POINT CODE

The vast majority of breast cancers are detected by women themselves which is why it's so vital that we're breast aware. The Department of Health recommends following these five steps:

Know what's normal for you We're all different and so are our breasts – they come in all shapes and sizes. The key is knowing what is normal for you. The more familiar you are with how lumpy your breasts are, what shape they are and so on, the more likely you are to notice any changes.

Know what changes to look for Look for what's not right for you. This might be a dimpled or puckered area, a rash on or around the nipple, an inverted nipple, an obvious swelling, discharge from the nipple, a change in the size or shape of your breast or a swelling in your armpit or around your collarbone.

Check the look and feel of your breasts There is no rigid, set way to feel your breasts; you have to decide what you're comfortable with and what's convenient for you. Some women prefer to lie down, others find it easier to check their breasts in the shower or bath, using soapy hands that run over the skin more easily. It's also a good idea to get into the habit of looking at your breasts daily in the mirror – maybe while you're getting dressed in the morning.

Report any changes without delay If you discover a change in one of your breasts, book an appointment with your GP right away. And don't panic! Most breast changes aren't cancer and are nothing to worry about, but it really is better to be safe than sorry; the earlier any problems are detected the greater your chances of a complete cure.

Attend routine breast screening if you're over 50 Mammography is available to all women in the UK between the ages of 50 and 70.

START CHECKING NOW

Obviously it's a good idea to check your own breasts, but I am sure your husband or partner would be more than happy to give them the once over and he probably knows them a lot better than you do! By going for help as soon as you spot any changes, you really can give yourself a fighting chance if it turns out that you do have cancer, but do bear in mind that it will more than likely be something minor like a cyst.

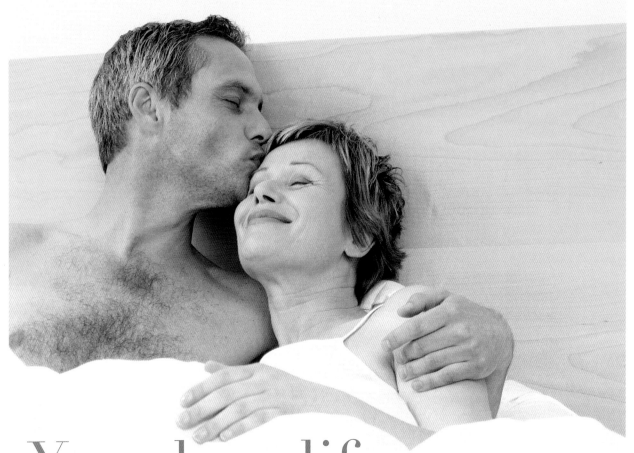

Your love life

AS WE GET OLDER, IT IS VERY EASY FOR OUR
SEX LIFE TO BE RIGHT DOWN AT THE BOTTOM
OF A VERY LONG LIST, PARTICULARLY FOR
THOSE OF US WHO'VE BEEN TOGETHER FOR A
WHILE AND THAT FIRST FLUSH OF INSATIABLE
LUST HAS DIMMED.

ike everything else that is worthwhile, you have to work at making love. Just because it was fantastic when you first started going out with each other, or before the kids came, doesn't mean it will stay that way forever. You need to make an effort to keep things fresh and exciting and never take each other for granted.

SEX IS GOOD FOR YOU

There's plenty of scientific evidence for the benefits that regular sex can have on your sense of wellbeing and on your health. We all know that it makes you feel happier and more relaxed, and it is a wonderful natural cure for insomnia. But there's more!

Studies have found that sexually active people live longer and take less time off work. And did you know that during orgasm your body produces phenetylamine, a natural chemical that controls your appetite? An extra bonus is that engaging in sex can also burn five calories a minute or more – great news for those of us trying to stay in shape.

From a health point of view, you produce testosterone when you orgasm, which helps protect your heart. Furthermore, having an orgasm will improve your circulation and boost levels of serotonin, which is vital for all-round good health.

MAKING TIME

Sex is a very important part of a loving relationship but often it gets put to one side as other areas of our lives take over. You may work long hours, have small kids, be stressed about paying the mortgage or perhaps you're just plain tired. Here are some ideas for getting that sexual sizzle back:

- 'Let's put it in the diary' sounds daft but, in fact, there's nothing wrong with scheduling a regular sex fixture. That way you can ensure that it actually happens, while the anticipation of it will keep you in a saucy mood all day.
- Being intimate doesn't always have to happen at night or at a weekend. A quickie in the morning may mean that you have to rush through your morning shower and make-up routine but looking a little less than perfect will be worth it!
- Plan for a hot date with your partner at least once a month. If you have children, gratefully accept all offers of babysitting and enjoy an evening that's just for the two of you. Candlelight, good food, a little wine. Who knows what it might lead to?

SEXUAL HEALTH

If you're in a new relationship or have more than one sexual partner, it is vital for your health that you practise safe sex and always use a condom. Sexually transmitted infections are unpleasant and can be life threatening. If you are at all worried that you may have a sexually transmitted infection, see your doctor or a clinic right away. And don't worry about what they'll think: they're there to help you and will be professional and non-judgemental.

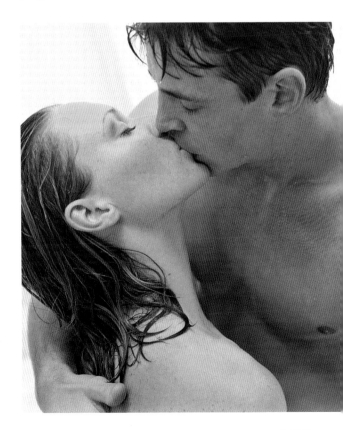

Look after your back

LIKE SO MANY PEOPLE, I HAVE SUFFERED FROM DREADFUL BACK PAIN – IN MY UPPER BACK, FROM HUNCHING OVER A COMPUTER SCREEN, AND ALSO DOWN MY RIGHT-HAND SIDE OWING TO THE SHEER WEIGHT OF MY HANDBAG! I FIND PILATES HAS SIGNIFICANTLY HELPED MY POSTURE.

ABOUT BACK PAIN

Around one in three people in the UK suffers from back pain at some point in their lives, mostly in the 35–55 age group. An astonishing 2.5 million of us see our GPs about back pain each year. And the numbers are going up in this computer age, with so many of us being guilty of slumping in front of our screens for too long.

Medically, back pain is classified as acute when the symptoms last for fewer than six weeks, or chronic when the symptoms last for more than three months. Luckily, most back pain is caused simply by the strains we put on our bodies and, if you stay active and take care of your back, it will heal itself. It's important, though, to see your GP to rule out any serious underlying causes, such as osteoarthritis or disc problems, if your back pain lasts for more than a week or two.

HOW TO PREVENT IT

There are some really straightforward things you can do to help ensure that you don't suffer back pain, such as:

Avoid being overweight This puts a strain on your back.

Reduce stress and tension Learn some simple relaxation techniques and use them regularly (see pages 176–77).

Take regular exercise Walking and swimming are excellent, as is Pilates, which is my favourite way of keeping in shape (see pages 90–117).

Lift and carry heavy things the correct way The step-by-step photos on the opposite page show you how to do it properly.

Check your posture Check yourself when you're standing and sitting, especially if you spend a lot of time sitting at a desk.

Avoid twisting back When you are picking up, reaching for or moving something, move your feet, turn your whole body and bend your knees rather than just twisting your upper body.

STANDING TALL

Do you know that you can look up to half a stone slimmer just by standing straight? Get into the regular habit of standing in front of a full-length mirror and running through this checklist to remind yourself about good posture:

- Is your head level, with your chin parallel to the floor?
- Is your back straight?
- Is your weight evenly distributed on both feet?
- Are your hips and shoulders level?
- Are your kneecaps pointing straight ahead?
- Are your hands relaxed and falling slightly in front of your thighs?

SITTING PRETTY

Remind yourself of these pointers to help you maintain perfect posture when sitting at your desk:

- Are your feet flat on the floor or on a foot rest? Try not to cross your legs as this tilts your pelvis too far forward and puts strain on your back.

- Are you sitting upright with support in the small of your back? You can use a little cushion or rolled-up towel to add support if you like.

- Are your knees and hips level?

- If you're using a keyboard, are your forearms, wrists and hands in a straight line?

LIFTING AND CARRYING

Think before you lift anything heavy, whether it's a toddler, a hefty box or an awkward chair. Can you manage it safely, how far are you planning to carry it and should you get someone to give you a hand? If in doubt, get help.

1 Your feet should be apart with one leg slightly forward to help you balance. Let your legs take the strain. You should bend from your knees but don't stoop. Try to tighten your stomach muscles to hold your pelvis in.

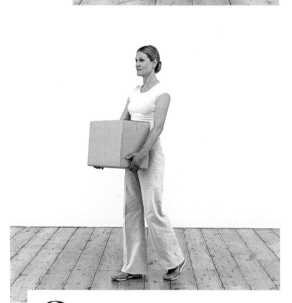

2 As you come up, lean forward slightly and keep your back straight. Remember not to straighten your legs before lifting the object, otherwise you might strain your back.

3 When you are holding the object securely, keep your head up and look ahead, not at what you're carrying. Hold the object close to your waist while you carry it and, when you put it down, repeat the sequence in reverse, remembering to bend from your knees.

Stay heart healthy

IN 1979 I DID A STORY ON THE BRITISH HEART FOUNDATION'S SEARCH FOR A 'QUEEN OF HEARTS'. THE CHARITY WANTED TO FIND A WOMAN WHO COULD RAISE AWARENESS OF HEART DISEASE, WHICH, EVEN THEN, WAS ATTACKING ALMOST AS MANY WOMEN AS MEN.

I found myself shocked at the scale of heart disease and volunteered to be one of the contestants. I was delighted to go on to win the title, partly through fundraising by embarking on a 50-mile (80 km) sponsored rollerskate from the 'heart' of East Kilbride to the 'heart' of Midlothian in Edinburgh.

It has meant a long association with the charity and a real desire to make sure that, in particular, women know of the dangers of heart disease – it's not just overweight, stressed-out businessmen who succumb to this widespread disease. The good news, however, is that you can take steps to protect yourself and your family.

THE FACTS

We tend to think of heart disease as a male problem but the reality is that almost as many women are affected as men. Over 100,000 women in the UK have a heart attack every year and, in the US, heart disease and stroke are the number one causes of death among women. Heart disease happens when the arteries in the heart itself become narrowed or blocked because of a build-up of fatty deposits. When nutrient-rich blood can't reach parts of the heart because of the narrowed and blocked arteries, the muscle tissue is 'starved' of oxygen and the result is chest pain (known as angina) or, in the worst case, a heart attack.

WHO'S AT RISK?

A number of factors influence the incidence of heart disease, including age. You are also more at risk if:
- There is a family history of heart disease.
- You have diabetes.
- You smoke, lead a sedentary life or eat a bad diet.
- You have high blood pressure or high levels of cholesterol.
- You are an 'apple' shape, meaning that you carry fat around your middle. People who are 'pear' shape – those who carry fat on their hips – are less likely to develop heart disease.

BE KIND TO YOUR HEART

There are some things you can't do anything about – like getting older or your family history – but there are plenty of things that you can do something about, and which will reduce your risk of developing heart disease:

Get active Exercise is absolutely essential for a healthy heart. Your heart is a muscle and, like any other muscle, it can be trained to become strong so that it can pump more blood with each heartbeat.

Enjoy a healthy diet There is plenty of evidence that links heart disease to a poor diet. As a guideline, you need to think less salt, less saturated fat and more fruit, vegetables and fibre.

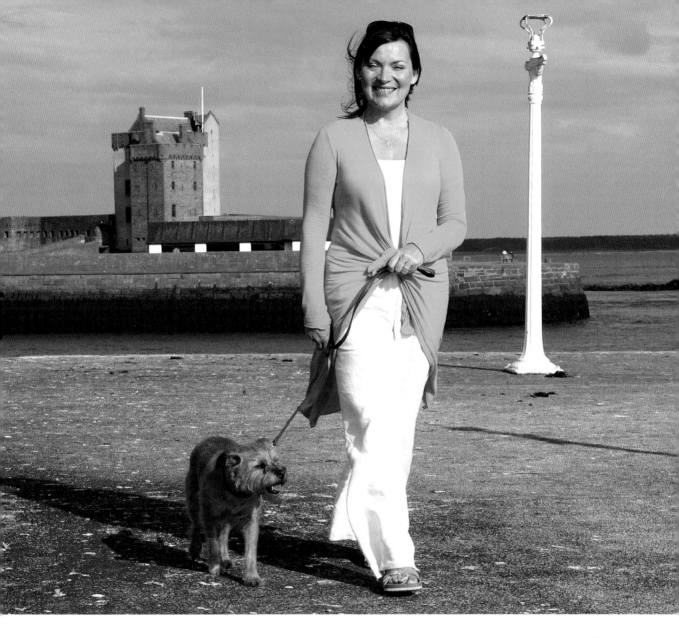

This doesn't mean a life without potato crisps or cakes; it just means that we should all aim to eat well most of the time (see Chapter 1: Healthy Eating).

Quit smoking Giving up will significantly reduce your risk of heart attack and stroke.

Drink in moderation People who drink too much are more likely to die of heart disease than those who don't (see pages 172–73).

Control cholesterol Cholesterol is vital for the human body but too much low-density lipoprotein (LDL) or 'bad' cholesterol adds to your risk of heart disease. Foods that are high in saturated fat, such as fatty meats, butter, cheese, cream, pastries, cakes and biscuits, will increase levels of LDL cholesterol, so you need to cut right back on these to protect your heart.

Keep your weight down You run an increased risk if you're overweight. Keep your weight at a healthy level or, if you're overweight, plan to lose the excess. You may want to try my personal Weight-loss Plan, which starts on page 36.

Healthy bones

I STOPPED YO-YO DIETING WHEN I REALIZED I
WAS STORING UP REAL TROUBLE FOR MYSELF
IN LATER LIFE, PARTICULARLY BECAUSE OF
THE INCREASED RISK OF DEVELOPING
OSTEOPOROSIS. A FADDY DIET ISN'T WORTH
THE EFFECT IT COULD HAVE ON YOUR BONES.

WHAT IS OSTEOPOROSIS?

It's a condition where the bones get thin and weak
and break easily. Our bones lose their strength and
density as part of the natural ageing process but,
for some of us, bone is lost faster than new bone
can be formed to replace it and when this happens
bones become very fragile.

Around three million people in the UK have
osteoporosis and it causes around 200,000
fractures each year. However, because the
condition is generally painless in the early stages,
you probably won't know if you have osteoporosis
until you actually break a bone.

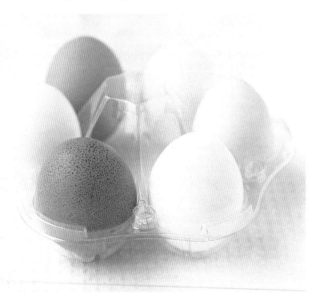

Some people are at higher than average risk of
osteoporosis and it's important to talk to your
doctor if you are concerned. You may have a greater
risk if, among other things, you have an early
menopause, have taken steroids for more than six
months, have a family history of the condition,
suffer from chronic illness, or if your periods have
ever stopped for a long time. There is hope, though!
Osteoporosis is not inevitable and could be avoided
if you eat the right diet, make good lifestyle choices
and do weight-bearing exercises.

FOOD FOR BONES

Calcium is a major component of the structure of
bones, so make sure that you eat plenty of foods
that are rich in calcium. A daily dose of 700 mg is
recommended and this should be pushed up to
1,200 mg during and after the menopause. We tend
to think of milk when we think of where to find
calcium but, amazingly, watercress and almonds
pack more calcium per 100 g (3½ oz) than milk!
This chart – which includes some surprises –
shows the calcium in 30 familiar products, to help
you make bone-friendly choices.

Fizzy drinks and caffeine can affect the calcium
balance in your body, so try to cut back on colas
and lattes and aim to swap one or two a day for
water or herbal tea. A diet that is too high in salt
also weakens bones, so think twice before you
reach for the saltcellar.

SOURCES OF CALCIUM

Food	Calcium (mg) per 100 g (3½ oz)
Cheddar	721
Camembert	288
Soya beans	277
Almonds	266
Watercress	192
Brazil nuts	176
Broccoli	123
Natural yogurt	121
Milk	119
Sunflower seeds	116
Spinach	101
Cottage cheese	60
Swede	58
Eggs	56
Oats	55
Green beans	48
Cabbage	47
Carrots	40
Oranges	40
Figs	35
Kidney beans	28
Raspberries	22
Chicken	16
Aubergines	12
Brown rice	11
Cod	10
Lamb	9
Salmon	8
Potato	7

IMPROVING YOUR LIFESTYLE

Smoking increases your risk of osteoporosis, which is yet another reason to give up. It's wise to limit your alcohol intake, too, as alcohol inhibits calcium absorption. And get some sun! Sunlight will trigger the production of vitamin D, which leads to your body absorbing more calcium. Don't overdo it,

though – 20 minutes of ultraviolet (UV) light a day in summer is all you need to supply your vitamin D needs for the year. Stay out of the sun when it is at its strongest, between 11 am and 3 pm (see pages 122–123). If you don't want to expose your skin to too much sunlight, consider taking a vitamin D supplement. Vitamin D is also available in small amounts in foods such as oily fish, egg yolks and liver and is added to some cereals.

SHAKE THOSE BONES

To strengthen your bones you should aim to do some weight-bearing exercise for half an hour at least three times a week. Good choices include walking, running, aerobics, tennis, weight-training, dancing and skipping. Even getting out into your garden and doing some digging or carrying a basket around the supermarket, rather than pushing a trolley, counts as weight-bearing exercise and it all helps.

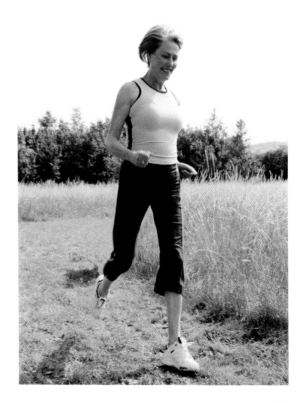

Alcohol awareness

ONE OF THE MOST DISTURBING MODERN
TRENDS IS THE RISE OF THE BINGE-
DRINKING FEMALE. GETTING SO DRUNK
THAT YOU FALL OVER IS NOT BIG AND IT'S
NOT CLEVER. A DRUNKEN WOMAN IS
VULNERABLE AND PUTS HERSELF IN A
VERY UNSAFE SITUATION INDEED.

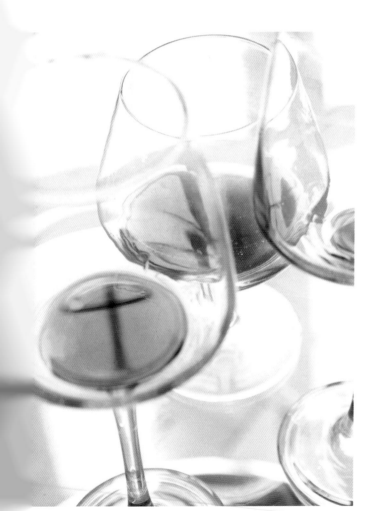

boozing also has disastrous effects on your looks and your health. I am obviously not saying don't ever have a drink. I'm partial to a glass of wine with my meal or a social drink with friends, but you need to know where to draw the line.

THE BAD NEWS

Drinking too much can lead to a number of serious health problems, including increased risk of liver disease, heart disease (see pages 168–69), osteoporosis (see pages 170–71), depression, raised blood pressure and a variety of cancers.

Another thing to remember is that alcohol can be fattening. At seven calories per gram it is just behind fat which contains nine calories per gram. There are 120 calories in a small gin and tonic – more than you'll find in some of your favourite chocolate bars.

THE GOOD NEWS

No-one is suggesting that we all stop drinking altogether and, in fact, various studies suggest that drinking in moderation can protect against heart disease and heart attack. Drinking too much, on the other hand, will have the opposite effect.

WINE (RED, WHITE, ROSÉ AND SPARKLING)

% ABV	small glass (125 ml)	standard glass (175 ml)	large glass (250 ml)
10%	1.25 units	1.75 units	2.5 units
12%	1.5 units	2.1 units	3 units
14%	1.75 units	2.5 units	3.5 units

BEER, LAGER AND CIDER

% ABV	½ pint	330 ml bottle	pint
4%	1.1 units	1.3 units	2.3 units
5%	1.4 units	1.7 units	2.8 units
6%	1.7 units	2 units	3.4 units

SPIRITS (GIN, RUM, VODKA AND WHISKY)

% ABV	small measure (25 ml)	large measure (35 ml)	double measure (50 ml)
38–40%	1 unit	1.4 units	2 units

HOW MUCH IS SAFE?

Current recommendations from the Department of Health are that men drink no more than 3–4 units of alcohol a day and women no more than 2–3 units per day.

Women have a lower limit because we tend to be smaller in build and also because our bodies contain less water which means that the alcohol we drink is less diluted and we don't process it as effectively.

KNOW YOUR UNITS

One unit is 10 ml or 8 g of pure alcohol. The number of units in any type of drink is based on the strength of the alcohol content and the volume of the drink.

The units in your chosen tipple can vary more than you would think. A glass of wine, for example, can have anything from just over one unit to more than three, depending on the strength of the wine and the size of the glass.

NO-ONE IS SUGGESTING THAT WE STOP DRINKING ALTOGETHER, BUT YOU SHOULD BE SENSIBLE AND NOT DRINK MORE THAN 2–3 UNITS PER DAY

To work out how many units there are in a drink you multiply the volume in millilitres (ml) by the strength of the alcohol (ABV) – which is normally printed on bottle label – and then divide by 1,000. The table above gives a guideline and will save you whipping out a calculator every time you have drink!

SENSIBLE DRINKING

If you think that you need to cut down on how much you drink, there are lots of ways to help. Try using a smaller glass if you are drinking at home and, when you're out, opt for a small glass of wine or a single measure of spirits. Pace yourself by drinking lots of water and make every second drink a soft drink.

Try not to drink alcohol during the week and, if you do overdo it one evening, follow this with a few days without alcohol to give your body a chance to recover.

Stop smoking

THERE IS ONE THING THAT I WOULD URGE YOU TO DO TO LOOK YOUNGER, FEEL BETTER AND LIVE LONGER AND THAT IS TO THROW AWAY YOUR CIGARETTES. I AM LUCKY THAT I NEVER SMOKED. I DID TRY ONCE IN THE BACK OF THE SCHOOL BUS WHEN I WAS ABOUT 13 BUT I NEVER REPEATED THE EXPERIENCE.

I am well aware of how tough it is to kick the habit, but I hope that smoking will become 'uncool' and that its unpopularity will encourage people not to start in the first place. I despair at the number of young women who still

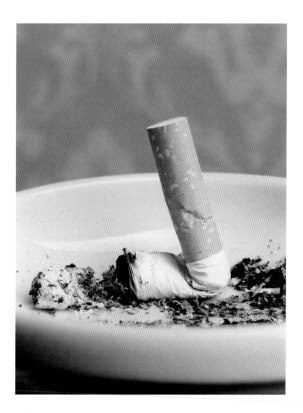

think smoking looks 'sophisticated' and who think that it will also keep them thin. Instead, smoking will give you a host of health problems and reduce your life span.

I was thrilled when the smoking ban came into effect, first of all in Scotland and then the rest of the country. I used to hate going for a meal and having to put up with smoke from other diners' cigarettes. The smell in my hair and on my clothes after a night in a smoky pub or bar was also horrible. Smokers themselves have become immune to the stench of stale smoke, but it really is a most unattractive pong.

WHY YOU SHOULD STOP

There are dozens of really good reasons to quit smoking; here are just some of the benefits you'll gain if you stub out that cigarette:

- You'll dramatically reduce your risk of developing cancer, heart or lung disease.
- You will save loads of money. Smoking 20 a day over a year costs more than a luxury, tropical-island holiday!
- You'll have increased life expectancy. Smokers die 10 years younger on average. The good news, though, is that quitting at any age will put years back on your life.
- You'll protect your family and friends from the

very real dangers of second-hand smoke.

- Your fertility levels will improve and you are far more likely to have a healthy pregnancy and a healthy baby.
- Smoking when you're pregnant is linked with an increased risk of miscarriage and can cause low birth weight and premature birth.
- You won't smell horrible.
- Your skin will get its glow and elasticity back and your teeth and fingers won't be stained nicotine yellow.
- Your circulation will improve and you'll have more energy and improved fitness.
- You'll be able to breathe more easily and you'll be able to enjoy the taste of food more.
- You won't have the anxiety smokers suffer when they have to spend a long time in a place where they aren't allowed to smoke, such as on an aeroplane.

GETTING HELP TO STOP

Quitting smoking is a hard thing to do and you are four times more likely to be successful if you have help when you decide to stop smoking, rather than trying to grit your teeth and go 'cold turkey'. Luckily there is plenty of help available, including:

Support There are many organizations, both local and national, that offer tremendous practical support in the form of booklets, e-mails, group meetings, telephone helplines and online advice. One of the best is the NHS Stop Smoking Service, which includes valuable advice from ex-smokers about how they managed to beat the habit. And, obviously, the more encouragement and motivation you get from family, friends and colleagues the better. Tell them that you're giving up and they'll be delighted to do all they can to help you.

Nicotine replacement therapy (NRT) This helps you get through withdrawal symptoms by supplying your body with a small amount of nicotine. Products are available over the counter or on prescription in the form of gum, patches, tablets, inhalers and nasal spray.

Prescription drugs If you really commit to

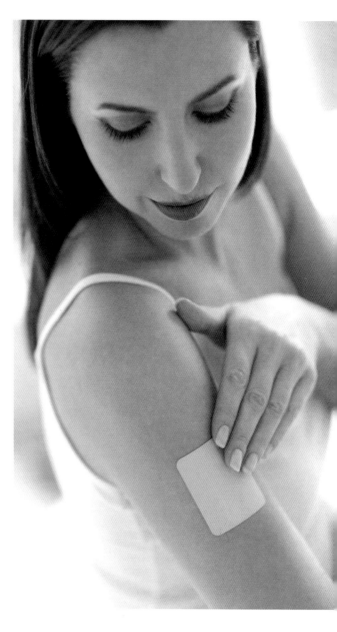

giving up, your doctor can prescribe drugs that will make you feel less like smoking and ease withdrawal symptoms. They're not suitable for everyone but it is worth speaking to your GP to find out more.

Complementary therapies There's no hard scientific evidence, but many successful ex-smokers swear by hypnosis or acupuncture and, if it worked for them, it may work for you.

Learn to relax

SO MANY OF US RUSH AROUND LIKE LITTLE HAMSTERS ON VERY BIG WHEELS AND WE BECOME MORE AND MORE WOUND UP AS EACH DAY GOES ON. WE NEED TO CHILL OUT! IT'S IMPORTANT TO PRIORITIZE – DON'T GET SIDETRACKED BY TRIVIA AND DON'T BE A SLAVE TO YOUR LAPTOP OR MOBILE PHONE.

SOOTHE AND CALM

Building time for relaxation into your life allows both your mind and your body to recover from the stress and rush of everyday life. Often something simple like curling up on the sofa to watch *Eastenders* or spending half an hour digging in the garden will do the trick, but sometimes you need to do a little more to relax properly.

There are relaxation techniques both for the mind and for the body, and using a mixture of both brings balance to your life and a sense of wellbeing. Here are some options you might like to try:

Meditation Although it takes practice, learning to meditate can help you to be more serene and self-confident, and that's not all. Clinical tests have shown that meditation has major health benefits – it can lower blood pressure, boost your immune system, ease pain and reduce muscular tension.

Yoga Yoga is a gentle exercise system that is good for both body and spirit. Stretching is the most natural way to release tension in your muscles and, combined with correct breathing as it is in yoga, relieves stress of the nervous system and increases energy levels so that you feel both calm and invigorated.

Reflexology In reflexology, specific points on the feet correspond to specific organs and systems in the body. Reflexologists can manipulate pressure points on your feet to counteract stress and to bolster your body's immune system. A good treatment is deeply relaxing and allows tension to ebb out of your entire body.

Massage Massage has been practised for thousands of years and is renowned for restoring physical and emotional harmony. Touch has been shown to increase the level of oxytocin, the hormone that makes us relax, in our bodies, making us calmer and healthier.

Aromatherapy Aromatherapy uses natural oils, such as lavender, neroli, ylang-ylang and rose, to heal both mind and body, and is good for reducing stress and aiding relaxation. The main way of using the oils is through massage and the wonderful smell of the essential oils, together with the effect of the massage as they are rubbed into your body, eases tension and brings a sense of total tranquillity.

> MAKE TIME FOR YOURSELF, EVEN IF IT IS ONLY FIVE MINUTES TO FLICK THROUGH A GLOSSY MAGAZINE OR CALL A FRIEND FOR A CHAT

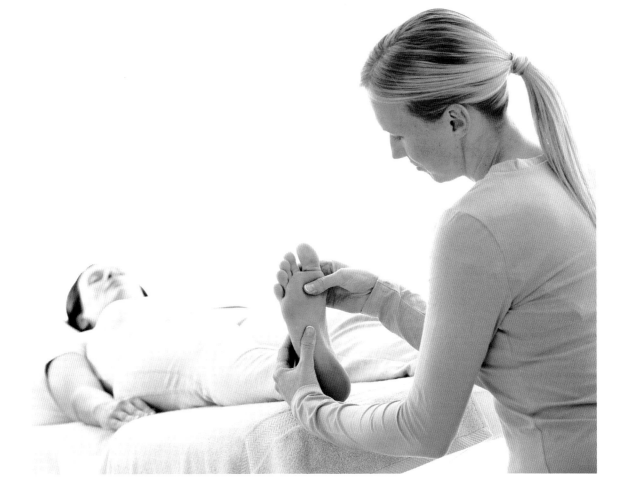

DEEP BREATHING

This easy exercise creates a deeper, slower breathing rhythm which, in turn, slows your heart rate and helps you to relax. It's most effective if you do it regularly, preferably twice a day, but it's also a handy soother when you're in a stressful situation – you don't have to lie down.

Begin by lying down on the floor and placing your hands on your abdomen, fingertips touching. Take a long, slow breath in through your nose as you count to five. Your lungs and abdomen will expand, which will make your fingertips part. Hold the deep breath for a count of five.

Very slowly, for a count of ten, breathe out through your mouth. You will feel your fingertips touching again. Keep on going, as though you are trying to empty your body of air completely. Repeat the whole sequence up to ten times.

MY TOP WAYS TO RELAX

- Taking my dog for a walk.
- Putting on a favourite dance tune and leaping around the room. In my case it's *I Predict a Riot* by the Kaiser Chiefs or *I Don't Feel Like Dancin'* by the Scissor Sisters.
- Reading a book by Maeve Binchy.
- Going on line to YouTube and looking at the sea otters that hold hands.
- Watching an old Hollywood musical – *Singin' in the Rain* does it for me.
- Watching reruns of sitcoms like *Frasier* on TV – laughter is such a good stress buster.
- Heading to my nearest beach and going paddling (bracing even in summer).
- Cuddling the ones I love.

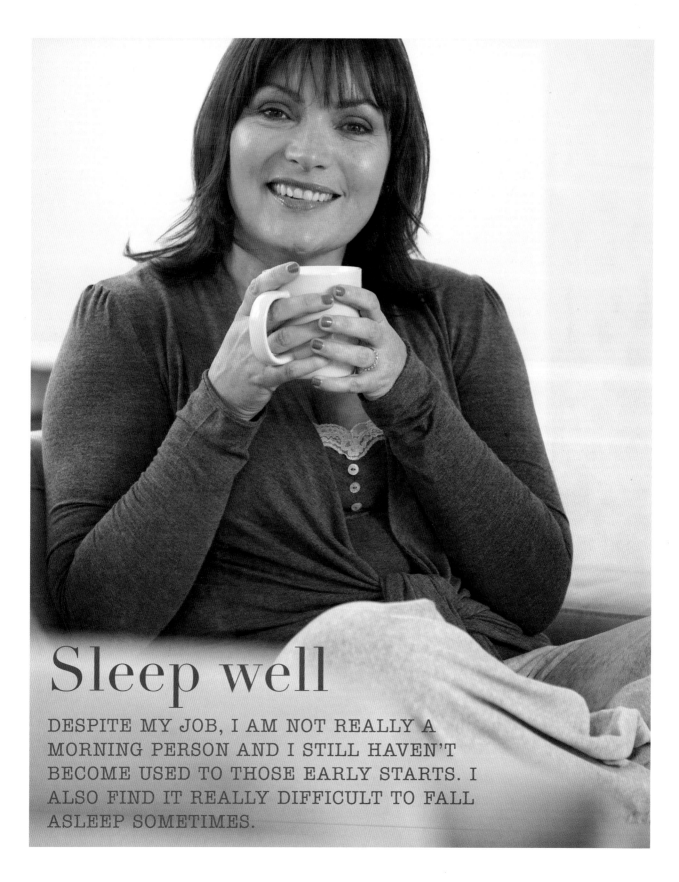

Sleep well

DESPITE MY JOB, I AM NOT REALLY A
MORNING PERSON AND I STILL HAVEN'T
BECOME USED TO THOSE EARLY STARTS. I
ALSO FIND IT REALLY DIFFICULT TO FALL
ASLEEP SOMETIMES.

W
hen I can't sleep, I don't lie there tossing and turning. I get up and run a bath with relaxing oils and maybe light some aromatherapy relaxation candles. I try to clear my mind of all the worries and concerns of the day and, if that doesn't work, as a last resort I change the sheets. There is something about freshly laundered bed linen that makes me sleep brilliantly.

WHY YOU NEED SLEEP

How much sleep you each need changes as you go through life and varies from person to person, but one thing is certain: we all need it. Getting a good night's sleep is vital for your health; it's how your body recharges itself and you need it for your brain to function properly.

Not sleeping can cause stress, high blood pressure and, some studies claim, can even lead to obesity. When you sleep your immune system becomes more active so, if you aren't sleeping properly, it doesn't function as well and it's harder for you to fight off illness. Lack of sleep shows on your face, too. Dark circles, saggy eyelids and a pasty complexion are signs that someone has had bad night.

Unfortunately, lack of sleep is one of the most common 21st-century health complaints; most of us have bouts of insomnia at times in our lives. There are a number of tricks you can try in order to get a better night's sleep naturally (I've suggested a few tips below), but if your insomnia goes on for an extended period, it's best to see your doctor about it.

TEN TIPS FOR A GOOD NIGHT'S SLEEP

1. A warm bath before bed stimulates the natural cooling process that the body uses to trigger sleep hormones. You'll add to the sedative effect if you put a drop or two of an essential oil, such as lavender or marjoram, in the bath water.
2. Your granny was right. A good, old-fashioned milky drink, such as a mug of warm milk mixed with a teaspoon of honey will help you get to sleep.

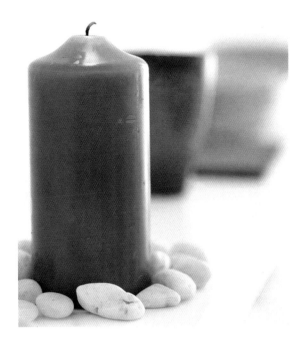

3. Including starchy carbohydrates, like brown rice, pasta or potatoes, in your evening meal may also help. These contain serotonin, which promotes relaxation and sleep.
4. Write down anything that is on your mind before you go to bed. That way your worries are on a piece of paper and not racing around your head.
5. Keep your bedroom as dark as possible. Light prevents melatonin from being produced, which is vital for helping our bodies recuperate.
6. A cool, well-ventilated bedroom (yes, even in winter) is best. Experts say that the optimum temperature for peaceful slumber is 18˚C (64˚F).
7. Try to plan your day so that you're tackling more taxing tasks in the morning and afternoon and aim to do more relaxing things in the evening.
8. Your bedroom should be a haven, not an entertainment centre! Keep the television, computer and stereo in other rooms.
9. Try to avoid caffeine, alcohol and nicotine for at least two hours before you go to bed.
10. Regular exercise is a great way to improve your sleep. Just be careful not to do it close to bedtime, as exercise produces stimulants that stop the brain from relaxing quickly.

Harnessing boundless energy

BEING TIRED ALL THE TIME (TATT) IS ONE OF THE HAZARDS OF MODERN LIFE AND 75 PER CENT OF US WILL SUFFER FROM IT AT SOME POINT. IT'S THAT HORRIBLE FEELING OF GOING TO BED EXHAUSTED AND WAKING UP FEELING WASHED OUT.

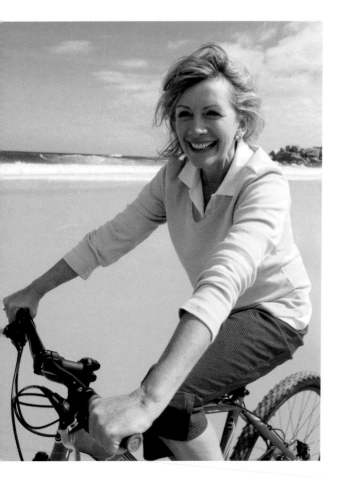

I have certainly experienced being TATT, especially when I was working as a TV news reporter and had such odd hours. If we were covering a main news story I might have to snatch a few hours' sleep in the car and grab food from all-night garages. At least I knew why I was exhausted and that when I got back into some sort of pattern, things would improve.

For so many women, however, being TATT becomes their norm. There are countless reasons for 'not firing on all cylinders' and, very often, just a few lifestyle changes will make all the difference.

GETTING YOUR BOUNCE BACK

If you feel that you need to recharge your batteries, there are some simple, but effective, lifestyle changes that you can make:

Eat well Check your diet for energy enemies, such as too much caffeine, junk food, ready meals and sugar. Try to eat regular meals, so that your body doesn't have to deal with energy-sapping sugar lows, and base your diet on whole grains, lean protein, fruit and vegetables. Breakfast really is the most important meal: you can set yourself up energy-wise for the day with a properly nutritious breakfast rather than shovelling down a hurried bowl of sugary cereal. See Chapter One: Healthy Eating.

Get enough sleep A good night's rest is the easiest and most natural way to reinvigorate yourself, yet an astonishing number of us don't get enough sleep. Only one in ten people in the UK gets the right quota – this varies according to individual needs, but is about 7–8 hours for most of us (see pages 178–79).

Exercise It may sound unlikely, but a walk will boost your energy levels more than a nap. Several studies have shown that even minimal regular physical exercise actually increases your energy levels rather than depleting them. (See Chapter Two: Exercise)

Drink plenty of water One of the most common reasons for low energy is not drinking enough water. Keep your fluid levels up by drinking little and often, and don't ignore thirst; that's a sign that your body needs more water. I always have a bottle of water in my handbag and I make an effort to drink 6–8 glasses a day.

Think right Nothing increases energy as much as enthusiasm. Often it's easier to focus on the negative things about our lives, rather than the positive ones, but this attitude is a huge drain on our energy.

Take time out This bit isn't easy if you have a busy career, hectic family life or both, but take time every a day to slow down for a while. Maybe make a cup of tea and sip it slowly, read a chapter of a book or just sit quietly for a few minutes in the car before you set off on the school run.

WHEN TO SEE YOUR DOCTOR

According to the *British Medical Journal*, for 90 per cent of us, illness is not the cause of fatigue. Sometimes, however, there is something more deep-rooted, such as anaemia or depression, underlying a lack of energy. Do go to your doctor if there are any other symptoms including nausea or loss of appetite or if you find that unexplained tiredness is seriously interfering with your day-to-day life.

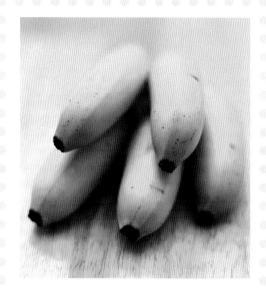

MY TOP ENERGY BOOSTERS

- Bananas: one of the best fruits ever and an instant energy giver.
- Nuts and raisins: a handful of almonds works really well for me.
- Smoothies: my favourite is mango and melon.
- Green tea: I make a big pot in the summer and stick it in the fridge. In the winter I sip a few small hot cups of it every day.
- Sushi: the Japanese know all about food that makes you feel energized and never bloated.
- Walking: preferably while listening to 80s' dance music.

EATING HEALTHY FOOD, DRINKING PLENTY OF WATER, TAKING REGULAR EXERCISE AND GETTING A GOOD NIGHT'S SLEEP WILL ALL HELP RECHARGE YOUR BATTERIES

Those hormones

HOW MANY TIMES HAVE YOU HEARD SOMEONE
SAY DISMISSIVELY ABOUT A WOMAN, 'OH, IT
WILL BE HER HORMONES' IF PERHAPS SHE
HAS BEEN A BIT SNIPPY OR TEARY?

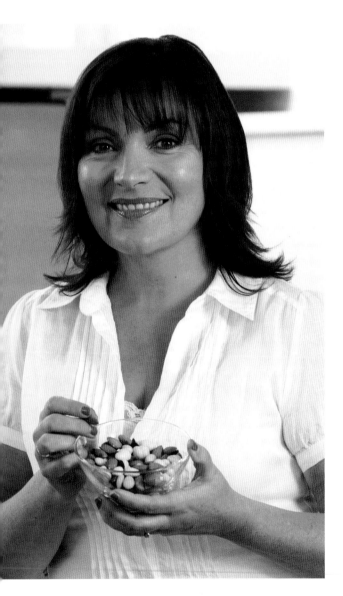

Very often a hormone imbalance can cause mood changes, especially before your period or before and during the menopause. Understanding what hormones are, what they do and how they affect you, can help deal with these changes to your body and to your emotions.

WHAT ARE HORMONES?

The word 'hormone' comes from the Greek *horman* meaning 'to stir up activity' and that's precisely what they do. From the day we're conceived, all through our lives, our bodies are under the influence of a cocktail of hormones.

Hormones are the body's chemical messengers; they travel around the bloodstream and act on tissues and cells. They are very powerful, each one acting on one type of tissue or cell only, controlling and activating functions. This system is very delicately balanced and if anything happens to disturb it, resulting in too much or too little of one hormone, the repercussions can be felt throughout the body.

Hormones play a big part in each woman's life, influencing moods, monthly periods, pregnancy and the menopause.

THAT TIME OF THE MONTH

Everyone's menstrual cycle is governed by hormones secreted by the endocrine system and many experts believe that premenstrual syndrome (PMS), is caused by an imbalance in hormones: too much oestrogen, prolactin and prostaglandins, and not enough progesterone.

Common symptoms of PMS are mood swings, irritability, spots, bloating, fatigue, breast tenderness and headaches. Many women also have a craving for sweets and chocolate.

BEATING PMS

When you're suffering from PMS you might feel that chocolate is the only answer, but you'll be wrong. In fact, many people think that the typical Western diet, with its high levels of sugar, salt, alcohol, caffeine and animal fat, is a key factor in rising levels of PMS.

Experts agree that the best diet for PMS – and for overall good health – is one based around starchy carbohydrates, with plenty of fruit and vegetables. It should also contain a little protein, some dairy foods and some unsaturated fat, found in seeds, nuts and oily fish. Cakes and pastries are best kept for an occasional treat. If you suffer from PMS, you should also try to cut back on alcohol and caffeine.

Exercise might seem the last thing you fancy when you have PMS, but it's worth it.

Several studies have proven that exercise can help to ease the symptoms. One study, for example, showed that regular running reduced breast tenderness, fluid retention, depression and stress.

WHEN YOU'RE PREGNANT

Hormones play a vital role in pregnancy, from enabling you to conceive in the first place to kick-starting contractions, and they're often blamed for the mood swings and tiredness that are common in pregnancy, too.

When you become pregnant a new hormone, human chorionic gonadotrophin (HCG) is produced by the developing placenta. This stimulates the ovaries to produce the higher levels of oestrogen and progesterone that you need. HCG is also the one to blame for morning sickness.

Oestrogen and progesterone are key players in pregnancy. Among other things, they cause the lining of the womb to thicken, increase blood circulation and prevent the uterine muscles from

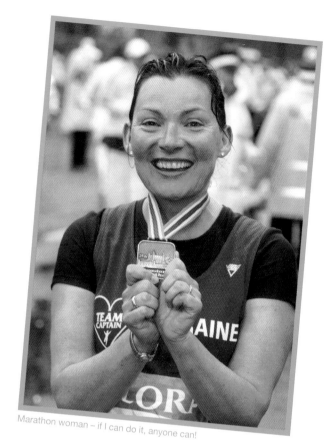
Marathon woman – if I can do it, anyone can!

contracting, so that your baby has room to grow. When it comes to the birth, other hormones play their part by helping the womb to contract during and after labour and by stimulating the production of breast milk.

HORMONES AND THE MENOPAUSE

The menopause happens when your ovaries no longer have a supply of eggs to release each month, as they did during your fertile years. One of the main hormones involved is oestrogen, which is produced by the ovaries themselves.

Around the age of 45, few eggs remain and the ovaries start to reduce their production of oestrogen, until it stops altogether during the menopausal years. During this time your body has to adapt to a life without oestrogen and that's what causes the menopausal symptoms many women go through (see also, pages 186–87).

Pregnancy

PREGNANCY IS ONE OF THE MOST IMPORTANT
TIMES IN YOUR LIFE FOR TRYING TO EAT
WELL AND DOING A SENSIBLE AMOUNT OF
EXERCISE TO ENSURE YOU GIVE YOUR BABY
THE BEST POSSIBLE START IN LIFE.

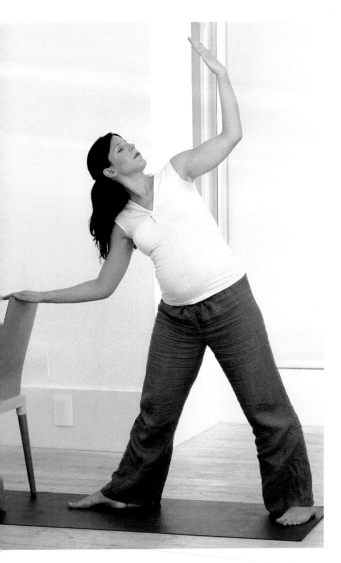

i absolutely loved being pregnant and I loved 'eating for two', which was very wrong of me. I was an Easter egg on legs and put on about four stone, most of which was down to fondant-filled chocolate eggs. Apart from those naughty eggs, I ate a really good diet of fresh fruit, vegetables and lean meat, but I just scoffed a bit too much, which made it so difficult to lose that baby fat later on. I also wish I had done more exercise because it would have been easier for me to get back into shape.

EAT WELL
A healthy diet is really important when you're pregnant or trying for a baby. Here's what you need to focus on:

Fruit and vegetables You need lots of these. Try to get in five portions a day, whether fresh, frozen or canned.

Starchy carbohydrates Foods such as breads, cereals, rice, pasta and potatoes should make up one-third of your daily calories. Choose wholegrain versions whenever you can.

Dairy products You need to eat 2–3 portions of these, which include milk, cheese and yogurt, each day.

Protein Found in things like meat, fish, poultry, eggs, beans, soya, pulses and nuts. Aim for a good variety and for about two portions a day.

Fats Your body needs good, unsaturated fats in the form of oily fish (for example, mackerel or sardines), olive oil and fresh nuts, and not the bad-for-you-fats that lurk in snacks, cakes and biscuits. You shouldn't eat more than two portions of oily fish a week, though.

THE DON'TS

Don't be tempted to 'eat for two', like I did. You don't need extra calories until the final three months, when you only need around 200 extra calories a day (that's about equal to two slices of buttered toast).

Pregnancy is really not the time to start dieting. This can affect your baby's weight, and may mean that you don't get the nutrients you both need. Don't skip meals, even if you feel sick; eating little and often can keep energy levels up and help to fight off morning sickness.

The government advises that you should avoid alcohol completely when you're pregnant. If you do drink, stick to no more than one or two units once or twice a week. I gave up booze altogether when I was pregnant and breastfeeding, as I didn't think it was worth the risk.

You should also be aware of the dangers for your growing baby if you smoke while you're pregnant, and should stop smoking for your baby's sake (see pages 174–75).

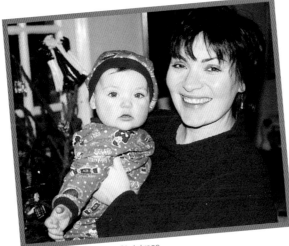

My angel – Rosie's first Christmas.

ENJOY YOURSELF!

Here are a few tips that were helpful for my own pregnancy and labour:

- Enjoy your pregnancy and don't let it stop you from your normal routine.
- Keep active and go for walks, but wear sensible shoes.
- It's OK to feel teary for no real reason during and after pregnancy, but if you feel really desperate seek help immediately.
- Have an open mind regarding your birth plan. If you want a natural birth that is fine, but don't rule out pain relief. There's nothing wrong with having an epidural. I had one myself and it was a blessing.
- Don't be afraid to ask your doctor and midwife questions.
- Try a TENS machine in the early stages of labour. It takes the edge off the contractions.
- The Queen's midwife told me that you should always keep your shoulders down during labour, as it instantly makes you relax. Simple but effective.

You don't need to cut out caffeine entirely, but shouldn't have more than 200 mg a day, which is roughly two cups of tea or instant coffee.

STAY ACTIVE

Gentle exercise will boost your feel-good factor, make you fitter and improve your strength and stamina, all of which are important to help you cope with the demands of pregnancy and labour. Generally, moderate, low-impact exercise is better than competitive sport – it's not advisable to push yourself too hard (see Chapter Two: Exercise).

Swimming and walking are good and yoga and Pilates are great too, so long as you stick to routines that are suitable for pregnancy. Look out for exercise classes for pregnant women at your local leisure centre or hospital. They're a terrific way of meeting other mums-to-be.

Facing the menopause

SO MANY WOMEN REGARD THE MENOPAUSE WITH HORROR AND DREAD, BUT I THINK WE WOMEN SHOULD JUST LOOK UPON IT AS THE NEXT NATURAL STAGE OF OUR LIVES AND ACTUALLY AS RATHER LIBERATING.

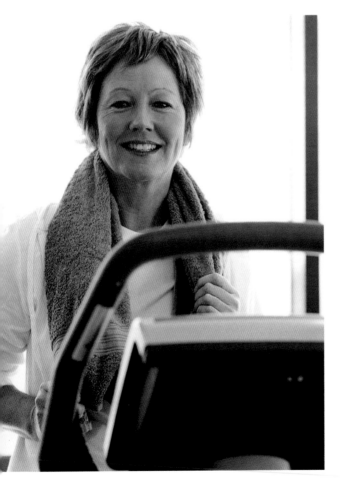

My mum sailed through 'the change' and I am hoping to do the same, but everyone is different. One thing you mustn't do is suffer in silence. Your GP has lots of treatments to alleviate symptoms so ask for help.

PERI-MENOPAUSE
This is the time leading up to the menopause and generally occurs around 3–4 years before your last menstrual period. This is when you notice the most significant physical changes, such as irregular periods and hot flushes.

MENOPAUSE
This is defined as your last period and the end of ovulation. In the UK the average age for a woman to reach the menopause is 52. It is generally considered to be over when a woman has not had a period for one year.

GETTING HELP
Reassuringly, over 90 per cent of women in the UK don't need to seek medical advice when they go through the menopause and many of those that do go to their doctor don't need any treatment at all, but if you are having symptoms that are really troublesome, there are treatments that can help.

COMMON SYMPTOMS

- **Changes to your periods** This is one of the earliest indicators. Your periods can become less frequent or more frequent, heavier or lighter.
- **Hot flushes** A hot flush is the feeling of heat that suddenly sweeps across the body. The skin on your face and neck might become red and you may start to sweat. It can last for anything from a few seconds to a few minutes and typically happens four or five times a day.
- **Night sweats** As the name suggests, these are hot flushes that happen at night, disturbing your sleep and drenching the bedding.
- **Insomnia** This can be caused by night sweats or general anxiety. You may find that the lack of sleep makes you grumpy or that you have trouble concentrating.
- **Vaginal symptoms** You may experience vaginal dryness, itching or discomfort.
- **Urinary symptoms** You might become more prone to urinary infections like cystitis and may need to go to the loo more often.
- **Mood swings and depression** Some women become moody and irritable and a few have feelings of low self-esteem.

Hormone replacement therapy is an effective treatment that replaces the oestrogen that naturally begins to decrease as you approach menopause, causing many common menopausal symptoms.

There are many different types of HRT and it comes in a variety of forms, including patches and pills. It's important to find the one that works for you.

As with all medication, there are both pros and cons to HRT and you should ask your doctor to discuss these with you. If HRT isn't suitable for you, your doctor may suggest alternative medication to help alleviate some of the symptoms, including antidepressants and medication to treat hot flushes.

THINK POSITIVE

Like many things in life, a positive outlook will help you to cope. Many women go through the menopause with few or no serious symptoms. No-one can predict exactly what will happen to you, but how you approach this new stage of your life will have a huge influence on how you deal with the changes going on in your body.

COPING WITH THE MENOPAUSE

Here are a few tips for getting you through the difficult days:

- Keep your bedroom cool and use cotton nightclothes and bed linen to ease night sweats.
- Dress in layers that can be removed easily if you get hot and put back on when you cool down.
- Try to steer clear of potential triggers like spicy food, caffeine and alcohol.
- Exercise regularly. This can improve hot flushes and combat mood swings and depression.
- When a hot flush starts, take slow, deep breaths.
- Running cool water over your wrists, spritzing your temples with cologne or putting a cool damp cloth on your forehead are all practical ways of easing a hot flush.

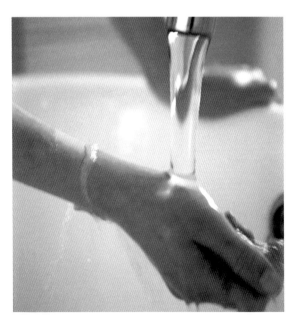

Love who you are

WORKING THROUGH THIS BOOK, YOU WILL
HAVE FOUND PLENTY OF ADVICE TO HELP
YOU TO GET INTO SHAPE, BUT THERE'S MORE
TO WELLBEING THAN DIET AND EXERCISE –
IT'S JUST AS IMPORTANT TO HAVE A SENSE
OF SELF-WORTH AND CONTENTMENT.

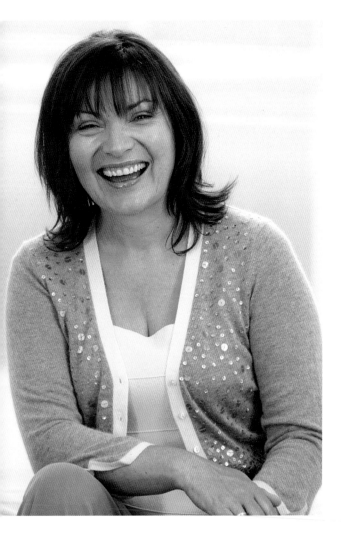

here is some invaluable advice to help you on your way to feeling positive about yourself and loving who you are.

DON'T STRIVE FOR PERFECTION

It is essential to acknowledge that nobody is perfect and neither should they try to be. Instead, remember that we are all unique and individual and – instead of aiming for an idealized perfection – you should value the woman you are and try to be the best version of *you* that you can be.

TAKE UP THE CHALLENGE

Don't be afraid to embrace new challenges and experiences. People who try different things and test themselves are happier than people who stick to familiar routines and activities. Bear in mind, though, that whenever you try something new, you're going to have to push yourself a bit. Losing weight or getting fit, for example, are not things that happen overnight.

THERE IS NO MAGIC PILL

You need to put in the effort. If you do, you *will* get results, but don't make things too hard for yourself by trying to do too much too soon. Please don't beat yourself up if, occasionally, you have a lapse. Instead, reward your successes and be proud of all that you achieve.

REWARD YOURSELF

It's important to reward yourself when you've done well and just as important to give yourself a treat for no other reason than that you deserve it! And you don't have to spend a fortune to enjoy a treat. Here are some of my favourites:

- Luxuriate in a candlelit bubble bath.
- Have an early night with a good book.
- Go for a massage, facial or manicure.
- Do something creative: take a pottery class or have a go at knitting a jumper.
- Pack a picnic and take the family to the park.
- Phone a close friend and enjoy a long chat.
- Treat yourself to a big bunch of flowers.
- Go for a cup of coffee in a local café and watch the world go by.
- Buy yourself a glossy magazine.
- Abandon the housework and watch your favourite TV show or an old black-and-white movie.

STAY CONFIDENT

We all have times of self-doubt or low self-esteem. Always remember that you are worthy of respect, and that what you think and say is just as important as anyone else's view or opinion. Remind yourself of these simple points when your confidence is at a low ebb:

DO:

- Believe in yourself
- Stick up for yourself
- Act confident, even if you don't really feel it
- Smile

DON'T:

- Dwell on negative things
- Surround yourself with people who are critical of you or sap your energy
- Frown

KEEP THE BALANCE

Sometimes it is fine to be a bit selfish. Creating 'me time' – time that is just for you, and has nothing to do with the demands of your job, your family or your home – is vital. Spending time on yourself and doing things that you enjoy, whether it's going to a weekly exercise or salsa class or a night out with the girls once a month, will give you something to look forward to. All areas of your life will benefit as a result.

LIVE FOR TODAY

My granny always said never keep anything for 'best', and nothing frustrated her more than women who left sexy lingerie unworn, still carefully wrapped in tissue paper in a bottom drawer, or never opened their favourite bottle of perfume. She said that you have to squeeze every drop of fun and happiness out of every single day. So, *please* don't put your life on hold until you have lost that stone in weight. You can still enjoy yourself while you are using this book to get yourself fit and healthy. Life is for living *now*, so get out there, grab it up by the scruff of the neck, give it a big, fat kiss and enjoy!

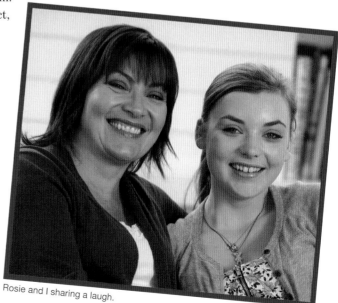
Rosie and I sharing a laugh.

Index

Acknowledgements

AUTHOR'S ACKNOWLEDGEMENTS

With thanks to my husband Steve, my daughter Rosie, Helen Hand, Mark Heyes, Jane Birch, Helen Foster, Jennifer Dufton and Sally Lewis.

PUBLISHER'S ACKNOWLEDGEMENTS

The Publisher would like to thank the following suppliers for sending us beauty products to use at the photo shoot. Body and nails: Jo Malone (www.jomalone.co.uk). Skincare: Liz Earle (uk.lizearle.com) and Origins (www.origins.co.uk). Make-up: Mac (www.maccosmetics.co.uk) and Bobbi Brown (www.bobbibrown.co.uk). The Publisher would also like to thank Marks and Spencers (www.marksandspencer.com) for lending us clothing and the Battersea branch of Powerhouse (www.powerhouse-fitness.co.uk) for lending us fitness equipment.

PICTURE ACKNOWLEDGEMENTS

All photographs are by **Russell Sadur**, with the exception of the following: **Alamy** Chris Rout 163. **Corbis** Frederic Cirou/PhotoAlto123; Ian Hooton/Science Photo Library 175; Lou Chardonnay 139; Michael A Keller 162. **Getty Images** Gazimal 42; Image Source 138; Ligia Botero 148; Louis Fox 180; Peter Dazeley 174; Stockbyte 17 above left. **Image Source** royalty free 164. Courtesy of **Lorraine Kelly** 15, 159, 183, 185. **Octopus Publishing Group** Emma Neish 11, 16; Frank Adam 29 right, 170; Gareth Sambridge 21, 26 left, 31; Ian Wallace 40, 179; Janine Hosegood 10; Jeremy Hopley 46; Karen Thomas 181; Lis Parsons 12 below right, 27 left & right, 29 left, 30 left & right, 32, 33, 44; Mike Prior 125, 167 left, above & below right; Peter Pugh-Cook 165, 184; Ruth Jenkinson 177; Sandra Lane 13; Sean Myers 38; Simon Smith 20; Stephen Conroy 48; Will Heap 26 right, 28; William Reavell 17 below right, 187. **Photolibrary** 171, Klaus Tiedge 186.

Executive Editor Jane McIntosh
Managing Editor Clare Churly
Senior Editor Fiona Robertson
Deputy Creative Director Karen Sawyer
Concept design Smith and Gilmour
Designer Janis Utton
Senior Production Controller Amanda Mackie
Photographer Russell Sadur
Stylist Mark Heyes
Hair and make-up Helen Hand and Hitoko Hombu
Picture Researcher Marian Sumega